KETO
DIET AFTER 50

How Ketogenic Can Help Over-50 Men and Women to Reset Metabolism, Lose Weight, Reverse Diseases, and Boost Energy. Including 20 Quick, Inexpensive, and Delicious Low-Carb Recipes

Maria Suzanne Stephens

Table of contents

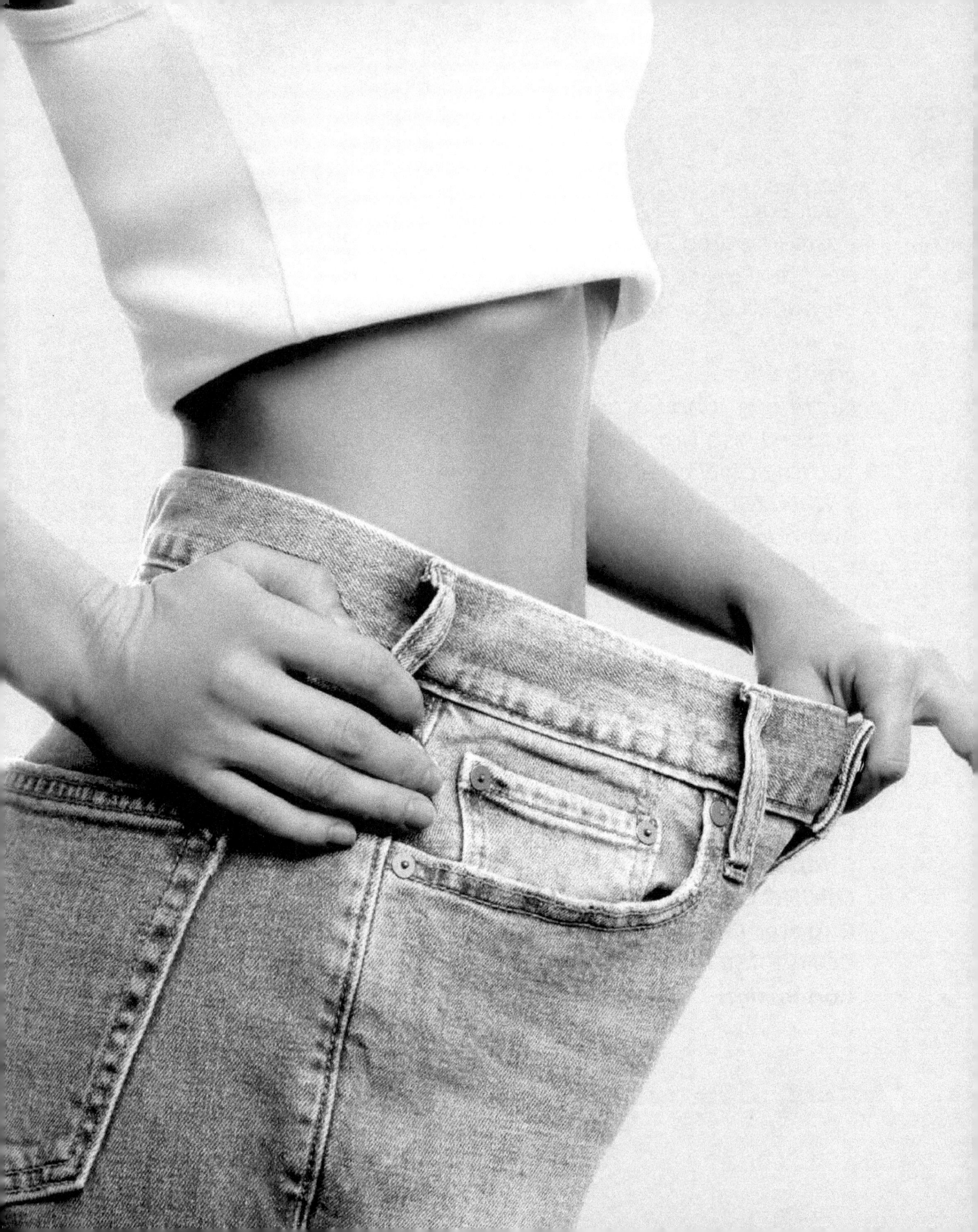

Introduction

This is a beginner's guide to successfully maintaining a Keto diet, as a woman or man over the age of 50-years-old. Over the last few years, you have likely heard a lot about the Keto diet. It is known as being a diet that allows you to indulge while still promoting weight loss. People of all ages have seen their incredible benefits.

The Keto diet consists of low-carb and high-fat food items which directly forces our body to burn all the fat for body energy in place of sugar and carbs. The keto diet forces our body to use up the stored fat, which allows the fat cells of the body to release all the fatty acids. The fatty acids, in turn, get converted into ketones by the liver. As soon as this process starts, the body gets into the state of ketosis, where ketones are burnt down for energy instead of sugar or glucose. As the overall intake of carbs gets reduced in this form of the diet, the ketones turn out to be the primary energy source. This ultimately results in a significant amount of weight loss.

A Ketogenic Diet is something that you should be starting with today for a better lifestyle if you are over the age of 50. The ketogenic diet is more common in women than in men because of all its benefits for dealing with the symptoms of menopause. Women who are experiencing menopause, or have already experienced it, have a clear idea of the troubles that come along with it.

The key to success is fueling your body correctly instead of stuffing it with overly processed junk. In this guide, you will learn everything you need to know from what to eat when to eat and how to get into the best shape of your life!

Packed with foods rich in protein and high in fat and doing away with carbohydrates is the ultimate way that the Keto diet helps you lose weight and maintain a healthy body. Instead of burning carbs, your body will be trained to burn fats, efficiently boosting your metabolism. It also turns your fats into ketones in your liver, which ends up providing you with additional energy for your brain.

Instead of focusing on the carbs that you will be giving up, the Keto diet aims its focus on all of the protein and fats that your body craves. There are many delicious recipes that you can follow and foods that you can eat, even when you aren't at home. The Keto diet is known for being one of the least restrictive diets, an essential aspect in helping you to follow through with it. This guide will answer all of the questions that you have about what the menu consists of and how to successfully make Keto a part of your daily life. Unlike other diets, you will be amazed at how much freedom you are still allowed. It is almost like you aren't even on a diet at all!

As your body and brain age, it is essential to pay attention to how you can successfully maintain your energy levels. Certain tasks become a lot more cumbersome when running on half the energy than you're used to. The Keto diet works very well for women, especially those over 50. Aside from the benefits to your metabolism and energy levels, you will also notice a decrease in inflammation, a stable blood sugar level, and balanced hormones. With all of these benefits in place, you will see that you will feel better both physically and mentally. And, of course, your mental health is very important to consider while on a diet. A lot of diets cause you to feel that you lack what you truly want to eat, therefore putting you into a negative mindset.

Keto is different, and this guide will show you all of the reasons why. It is an overall lifestyle change that is possible for almost everyone, no matter what your average day looks like. You will be filled with plenty of optimism and all of the positivity necessary to meet your goals. Whether you want to maintain your current weight or lose weight, Keto will help you get to where you truly want to be. It will become an anti-aging diet that will ultimately be a regular part of your everyday life.

If you are ready to feel great and look great, then you are ready to begin your own Keto diet. It will be a diet like no other because you will feel great every step of the way. There are no tricks or deceiving steps that you must take to succeed with the diet. As long as you are educated on what you need to be eating, you should have no problem incorporating the Keto diet into your current lifestyle.

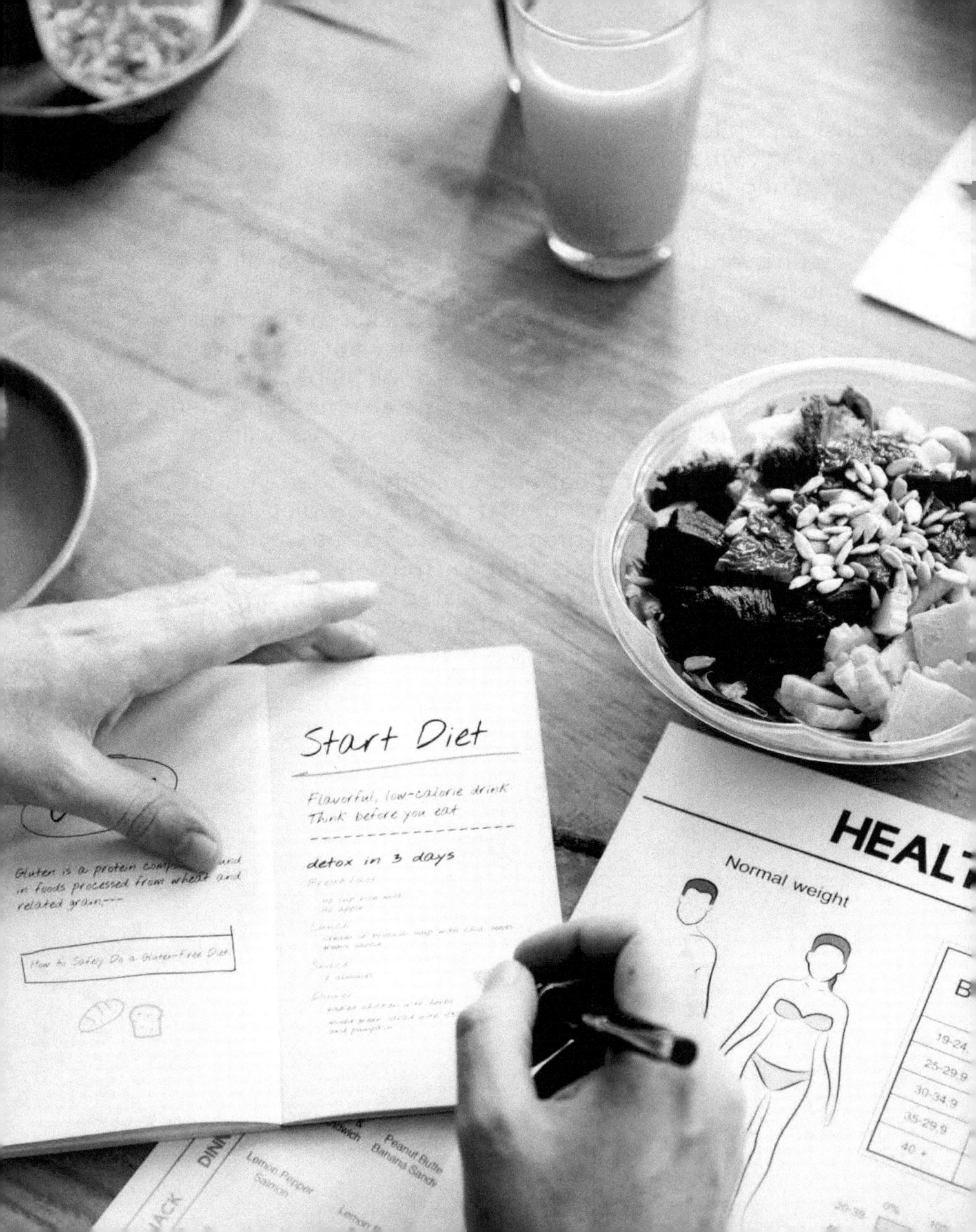

Start Diet

Flavorful, low-calorie drink
Think before you eat
- - - - - - - - - - - - - - -
detox in 3 days

Gluten is a protein confi... ...und
in foods processed from wheat and
related grain---

How to Safely Do a Gluten-Free Diet

HEALT

Normal weight

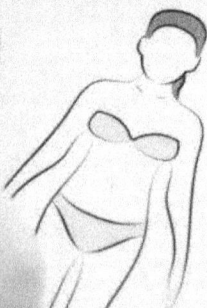

Chapter 01
What the Keto Diet Is and What It Is Not

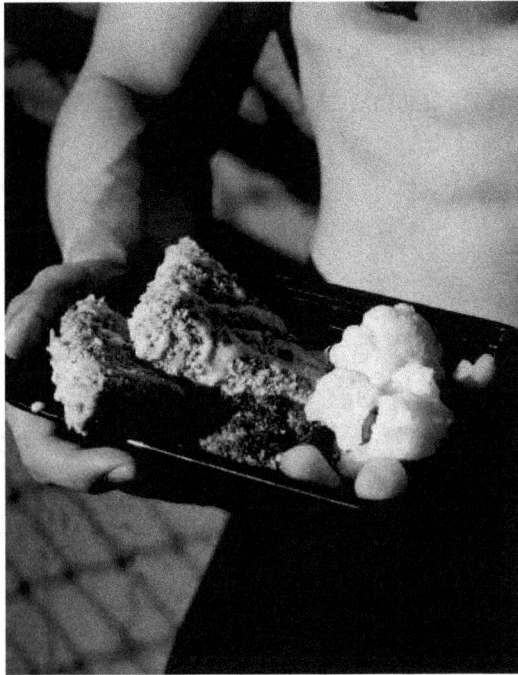

Keto is the short form of ketogenic. Keto is a low carbohydrate diet that is high in fats and uses an adequate amount of proteins. Our body needs energy to perform daily activities. These energies are consuming from food in the form of carbohydrates, fats, and proteins.

There are indeed countless diet plans out there on the market, and it would be too arrogant to say that the keto diet is the best among them all. However, it would be fair to say that the keto diet is the best one for you personally if it happens to serve your needs and goals more effectively.

The keto diet is a low-carb diet designed to put the human body into a heightened ketogenic state, which would inevitably lead to more pronounced fat burn and weight loss. It is a fairly accessible diet with many keto-friendly foods being readily available in marketplaces at relatively affordable prices. It isn't a diet that is reserved only for the affluent and elite.

As far as effectiveness is concerned, there is no denying how impactful a keto diet can be for a person who wants to lose a drastic amount of weight in a healthy and controlled manner. The keto diet also enforces discipline and precision for the agent by incorporating macro counting and food journaling to ensure accuracy and accountability in the diet. There are no external factors that can impact how effective this diet can be for you. Everything is all within your control.

And lastly, it's a fairly sustainable diet plan, given that it doesn't compromise on flavor or variety. Sure, there are plenty of restrictions. But ultimately, there are a lot of alternatives and workarounds that can help stave off cravings. If all these principles and reasons apply to you and your own life, then it would be safe to say that the keto diet is the best one.

HOW THE KETOGENIC DIET WORKS

Welcome to your first Ketogenic Diet Science lesson! One of the best parts of the Ketogenic Diet is that it is based on a natural process that your body already has!

The first lesson you need to know is that our body has four primary fuels that we use. These include glucose, protein, free fatty acids, and ketones. Each one of these fuel sources is stored in different proportions in our bodies. Overall, the fuel that we use the most is stored as triglyceride in our adipose tissue, aka, FAT! The second most used source is protein and glucose, used depending upon the metabolic state of your body.

So, what determines what fuel to use and when? As you might have already guessed, the primary determinant is based upon carbohydrate availability. Additional factors that can affect fuel utilization include a full or empty liver glycogen level and certain enzymes' levels. Overall, total energy equals glucose plus FFA.

Next, you must understand that the body has three different fuel storages that it taps into when you begin to lower your calories. These three different storage depots include protein, carbohydrates, and fats! Protein is essential in your diet because it can be converted into glucose in your liver and used as energy. Carbohydrates are typically stored as glycogen and are placed in your liver and muscle. On the other hand, fat is generally stored as body fat, but we will get to that in a second.

When you follow a SAD diet or a Standard American Diet, ketones truly have a nonexistent role in your energy production. However, as you begin a ketogenic diet, it will play a much more significant role. Here we introduce the fourth potential fuel source for your body! As you start to decrease the carbohydrate availability through diet, your body will automatically shift to using fat as your first fuel source.

PREPARING YOURSELF FOR KETO

When entering the keto world, quite a few of us just pick up a recipe on the internet and start cooking things accordingly. While that is good, we tend to search for any specifics which we should know of, such as what would happen if I replace nuts with something else? Is oatmeal a part of the keto diet? What are Keto approved food items? Are there any risks involved?

Here is some more information regarding such questions:

- Keto is an extremely strict food diet where you can only eat things that can be classified as Keto worthy. Anything that falls out of this category is a straight "no!"

- Keto is a completely new lifestyle. That means your body will undergo some changes. While most of these will be good, some may pose problems such as the keto flu.

- You will need to work on your cooking skills as Keto strictly pushes processed, high carb foods out of the diet.

- If you aren't really into the idea of protein and fat intake, you may wish to reconsider, as these are the two primary areas Keto focuses on.

Chapter 02

Why Keto Is Important

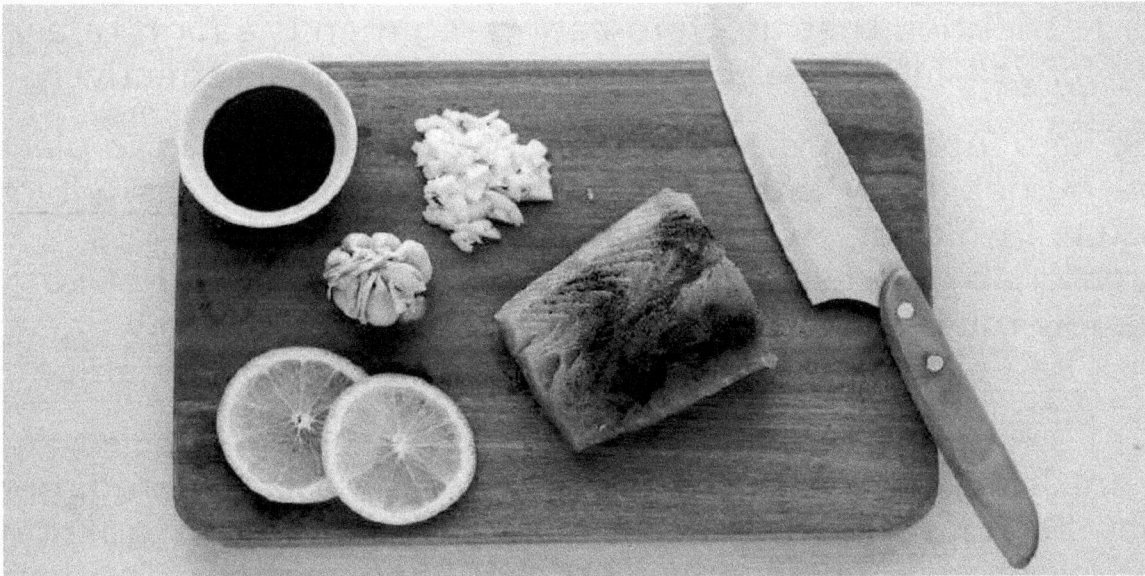

THE KETO DIET VERSUS OTHER LOW-CARB DIETS

Low-carb diets and the keto diet have been around for some time now, but as we've said, these two diets are different from each other. The effects they have on the body vary too; thus, you should know which type of diet you're following so you know exactly what foods to eat and avoid.

A low-carb diet involves eating minimal amounts of carbohydrates. The amount may differ from one diet to another. Still, the trouble with low-carb diets is that they don't consider the other types of macronutrients, such as proteins and fats. Conversely, the keto diet considers all the macronutrients in the equation, which gives your body an alternative source of fuel, which are the ketones. The great thing about the keto diet is that, unlike the other low-carb diets, you can measure your ketosis state. This allows you to know if the diet is working.

KETO AS THE BEST DIET PLAN OUT THERE

There are undoubtedly many weight loss plans obtainable on the market, and it'd be too arrogant to say that the keto weight loss plan is high-quality among them all. However, it would be fair to mention that the keto eating regimen is a high-quality one for you if it serves your wishes and your goals effectively.

The keto food plan is a low-carb diet that is designed to place the human body into a heightened ketogenic state, which results in higher pronounced fat burn and weight loss. It is a reasonably accessible food regimen with a variety of keto-friendly meals readily available in marketplaces at low prices. It isn't an eating regimen that is reserved only for the affluent and elite.

There is no denying how impactful a Keto eating regimen may be for someone who wants to lose a drastic quantity of weight in a wholesome and managed manner. The keto weight-reduction plan enforces discipline and precision by incorporating macro counting and meal journaling to ensure accuracy and accountability in the weight-reduction project

And lastly, it's a reasonably sustainable weight loss plan, for the reason that it doesn't merely compromise on taste or range. Sure, there are lots of restrictions. But ultimately, there are lots of alternatives and workarounds that can assist you to stave off cravings. If these kinds of standards and reasons work for you and your personal life, then it could genuinely be safe to say that the keto food plan is a right for you.

WHAT DISEASES CAN YOU PREVENT FOLLOWING KETO?

Heart Disease

As you begin to cut carbohydrates from your diet, it can help keep your blood glucose stable and low. By doing this, individuals have been able to keep their blood pressure in check. They are also able to lower their triglyceride levels.

When people first begin a Ketogenic Diet, they feel that it is counterintuitive to eat a higher percentage of fat to lower the triglycerides. Still, the truth is, fat has had a bad rep this whole time! It is eating excessive carbohydrates, especially fructose, that is the culprit behind increasing triglycerides! Through this new diet, you will be able to raise your good cholesterol and lower your bad cholesterol.

Fight Cancer

When it comes to cancer, you must seek medical attention before taking your life into your own hands through diet. It is highly advised that you listen to your doctor's advice regarding cancer treatment. However, there have been articles published based on cancer and the ketogenic diet showing that keto may help cure cancer.

Decrease Inflammation

Inflammation is a strange defense mechanism used in the body to help the immune system recognize any damaged cells, pathogens, or irritants. Through inflammation, the body can identify these issues and begin the healing process. While this is beneficial for the most part, unfortunately, it can persist longer than needed and will cause more harm than good. If you have inflammation in your body, you may experience symptoms such as pain, redness, swelling, immobility, and sometimes even heat. But, these signs of inflammations only apply to the inflammations on the skin. Sometimes, inflammation can happen within our internal organs. That is when we experience fever, abdominal pain, chest pain, mouth sores, and even fatigue.

Gastrointestinal and Gallbladder Health

If you suffer from heartburn or acid reflux daily, you may want to take a good, hard look at your diet. Unfortunately, many sugary foods, nightshade vegetables, and grain-based foods are major culprits of both heartburn and acid reflux. With that in mind, it shouldn't be a surprise that when you change your diet to include low-carb foods, these symptoms will disappear almost instantly. You experience these issues through an autoimmune response, bacterial issue, and inflammation caused by these foods in the first place.

Combats Metabolic Syndrome

As you grow older, you may find that you struggle to control your blood sugar level. Metabolic syndrome is another condition that has been proven to influence diabetes and heart disease development. The symptoms associated with metabolic syndrome include but are not limited to high triglycerides, obesity, high blood sugar level, and low levels of high-density lipoprotein cholesterol.

Fights Neurological Disorders

Keto diet has been used to treat neurological disorders or other cognitive impairments such as epilepsy. When your body goes into ketosis, your body produces ketones that help reverse neurodegenerative illnesses. Here, the brain just uses another source of energy instead of using the cellular energy pathway that is faulty in people with brain disorders. That means the keto diet can help prevent or treat disorders such as Parkinson's and Alzheimer's.

May Reduce Seizure Risk

When you change your intake levels of protein, fat, and carbs, as we explained before, your body will go into ketosis. Ketosis has been proven to reduce seizure levels in people who suffer from epilepsy. When they do not respond to treatment, the ketosis treatment is used. This has been done for decades.

Improved Kidney Function

Another common issue among the health community is kidney stones. The most common cause of both gout and kidney stones is due to elevated levels of phosphorus, oxalate, calcium, and uric acid in the body. Unfortunately, this is often combined with obesity, dehydration, bad genetics, sugar consumption, and alcohol consumption.

Reduces the Risk of Acne

You'd think a person in their 50's wouldn't have acne – and you'd probably be right. Note, though, that a large part of what you eat affects skin health, even if you're already in your 50s. People in their 50s need to be extra careful with skin health because this is when growths, blackheads, pore blockages, and more become persistent. Studies show that rapid changes in blood sugar affect skin health, as discussed in a study titled: Nutrition and acne – the therapeutic potential of ketogenic diets.

May Help Reduce Cancer Risks

Switching to the Ketogenic Diet may help reduce the risk of cancer, especially as its risk increases upon reaching the age of 50. Although that's just a small percentage, it's worth noting – especially if you happen to have a history of cancer. It's also interesting to note that the Ketogenic Diet is usually prescribed as a complement to chemotherapy. A study titled "Ketogenic diets as adjuvant cancer therapy: history and potential mechanism" concluded that sugar deprivation causes more stress to the cancer cells. This simply means that cancer cells depend more on the glucose you have on your body, and once their energy source is cut-off, they're more likely to die off.

Reduces Risk of Heart Problems

The healthy fat found in avocado, nuts, and other food items promoted by the Ketogenic Diet can help reduce the possibility of heart problems. A study titled: The long-term effects of a ketogenic diet in obese patients shows that going on a Keto Diet significantly increases HDL and lowers LDL. HDL is known as "good cholesterol." At the same time, LDL is the "bad cholesterol" known for increasing the likelihood of heart problems. The bad type is still discouraged and is not part of the Ketogenic Diet.

Chapter 03

Keto Products

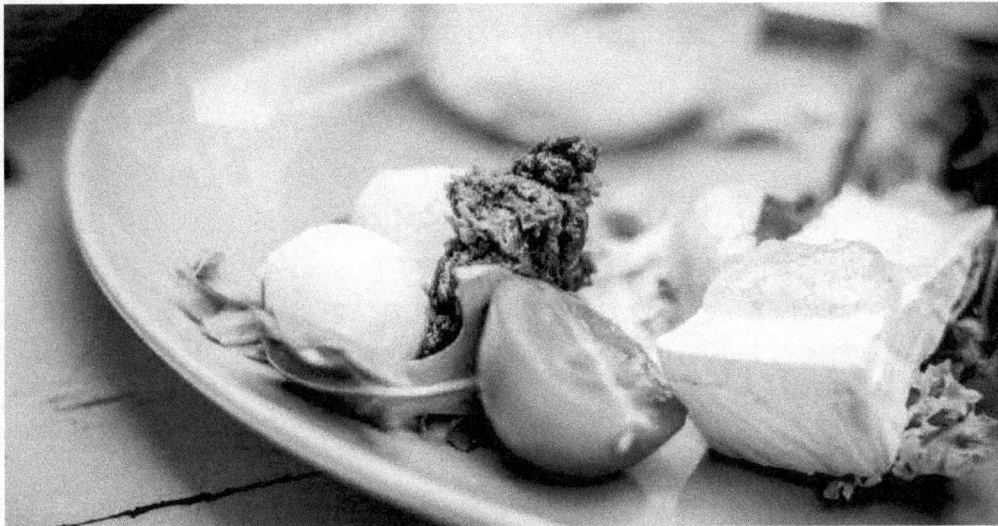

WHAT FOODS ARE ALLOWED

In this chapter, I will go over what food you should consider incorporating into your keto diet. But the general guideline is that all foods that are nutritious and low in carbs are excellent options.

Seafood

Fish and shellfish are perfect for keto diets. Many fish are rich in B vitamins, potassium, as well as selenium. Salmon, sardines, mackerel, and other fatty fish also pack a lot of omega-3 fats to regulate insulin levels. These are so low in carbs that it is negligible.

Shellfish is a different story because some contain very few carbs, whereas others pack plenty. Shrimp and most crabs are OK but beware of other types of shellfish.

Vegetables

Most vegetables pack a lot of nutrients that your body can greatly benefit from even though they are low in calories and carbs. Plus, some of them contain fiber, which helps with your bowel movement. Moreover, your body spends more energy breaking down and digesting food rich in fiber, which helps with weight loss.

Cheese

You can get away with cheese, as cheese is delicious and nutritious. Thankfully, although hundreds of types of cheese are out there, all of them are low in carbs and full of fat. Eating cheese may even help your muscles and slow down aging.

Avocados

Avocados are so famous nowadays in the health community that people associate the word "health" to avocados. This is for a very good reason because avocados are very healthy. They pack lots of vitamins and minerals, such as potassium. Moreover, avocados are shown to help the body go into ketosis faster.

Meat and Poultry

These two are the staple food in most keto diets. Most of the keto meals revolve around using these two ingredients. This is because they contain no carbs and pack plenty of vitamins and minerals. Moreover, they are a great source of protein.

Eggs

Eggs form the bulk of most food you will eat in a keto diet because they are the healthiest and most versatile food item of them all. Even a large egg contains so little carbs but packs plenty of protein, making it a perfect option for a keto diet.

Moreover, eggs are shown to have an appetite suppression effect, making you feel full for longer as well as regulating blood sugar levels. This leads to lower calorie intake for about a day. Just make sure to eat the entire egg because the nutrients are in the yolk.

Coconut Oil

Coconut oil and other coconut-related products such as coconut milk and coconut powder are perfect for a keto diet. Coconut oil, especially, contains MCTs converted into ketones by the liver to be used as an immediate source of energy.

Plain Greek Yogurt and Cottage Cheese

These two food items are rich in protein and a small number of carbs, small enough that you can safely include them into your keto diet. They also help suppress your appetite by making you feel full for longer, and they can be eaten alone and are still delicious.

Olive Oil

Olive oil is very beneficial for your heart because it contains oleic acid that helps decrease heart disease risk factors. Extra-virgin olive oil is also rich in antioxidants. The best thing is that olive oil can be a main source of fat and has no carbs. The same goes for olive.

Nuts and Seeds

These are also low in carbs but rich in fat. They are also healthy and have a lot of nutrients and fiber. They help reduce heart disease, cancer, depression, and other risks of diseases. The fiber in these also help make you feel full for longer, so you would consume fewer calories. Your body would spend more calories digesting them.

Berries

Many fruits pack too many carbs that make them unsuitable in a keto diet, but not berries. They are low in carbs and high in fiber. Some of the best berries to include in your diet are blackberries, blueberries, raspberries, and strawberries.

Butter and Cream

These two food items pack plenty of fat and a very small amount of carbs, making them a good option to include in your keto diet.

Unsweetened Coffee and Tea

These two drinks are carb-free, so long as you don't add sugar, milk, or any other sweeteners. Both contain caffeine that improves your metabolism and suppresses your appetite. A word of warning to those who love light coffee and tea lattes, though. They are made with non-fat milk and contain a lot of carbs.

WHAT IS NOT ALLOWED

Bread and Grains

Bread is a staple food in many countries. You have loaves, bagels, tortillas; the list goes on. However, no matter what form bread takes, they still pack a lot of carbs. The same applies to whole grain as well because they are made from refined flour. Grains such as rice, wheat, and oats pack a lot of carbs as well. So, limit or avoid that as well.

Fruits

Fruits are healthy for you. They have been linked to a lower risk of heart disease and cancer. However, there are a few that you need to avoid in your keto diets. The problem is that some of those foods pack quite a lot of carbs such as banana, raisins, dates, mango, and pear.

As a general rule, avoid sweet and dried fruits. Berries are an exception because they do not contain as much sugar and are rich in fiber. So, you can still eat some of them, around 50 grams. Moderation is key.

Vegetables

Vegetables are just as healthy for your body. Most of the keto diet does not care how many vegetables you eat so long as they are low in starch. Vegetables that are rich in fiber can help with weight loss. For one, they make you feel full for longer, so they help suppress your appetite. Another benefit is that your body would burn more calories to break and digest them. Moreover, they help control blood sugar and aid with your bowel movements.

But that also means you need to avoid or limit vegetables that are high in starch because they have more carbs than fiber. That includes corn, potato, sweet potato, and beets.

Pasta

Pasta is also a staple food in many countries. It is versatile and convenient. As with any other convenient food, pasta is rich in carbs. So, spaghetti or any other types of pasta are not recommended when you are on your keto diet. You can probably get away with it by eating a small portion, but that is often not possible.

Thankfully, that does not mean you need to give up on it altogether. If you are craving pasta, you can try some other alternatives low in carbs such as spiralized veggies or shirataki noodles.

Cereal

Cereal is also a huge offender because sugary breakfast cereals pack a lot of carbs. That also applies to "healthy cereals." Just because they use other words to describe their product does not mean that you should believe them. That also applies to oatmeal, whole-grain cereals, etc.

When you eat a bowl of cereal when you are doing Keto, you are already way over your carb limit, and we haven't even added milk into the equation! Therefore, avoid whole-grain cereal or cereals that we mention here altogether.

Beer

In reality, you can drink most alcoholic beverages in moderation without fear. For instance, dry wine does not have many carbs, and hard liquor has no carbs. So you can drink them without worry. Beer is an exception to this rule because it packs a lot of carbs.

Carbs in beers or other liquid are considered to be liquid carbs, and they are even more dangerous than solid carbs. You see, when you eat food that is rich in carbs, you at least feel full.

When you drink liquid carbs, you do not feel full as quickly, so the appetite suppression effect is little.

Sweetened Yogurt

Yogurt is very healthy because it is tasty and does not have that many carbs. It is a very versatile food to have in your keto diet. The problem comes when you consume yogurt variants rich in carbs such as fruit-flavored, low-fat, sweetened, or non-fat yogurt. A single serving of sweetened yogurt contains as many carbs as a single serving of dessert.

If you love yogurt, you can get away with half a cup of plain Greek yogurt with 50 grams of raspberries or blackberries.

Juice

Fruit juices are perhaps the worst beverage you can put into your system when you are on a keto diet. One may argue that juice provides some nutrients, but the problem is that it contains many carbs that are very easy to digest. As a result, your blood sugar level will spike whenever you drink it. That also applies to vegetable juice because of the fast-digesting carbs present.

Another problem is that the brain does not process liquid carbs the same way as solid carbs. Solid carbs can help suppress appetite, but liquid carbs will only put your appetite into overdrive.

Beans and Legumes

These are also very nutritious as they are rich in fiber. Research has shown that eating these have many health benefits, such as reduced inflammation and heart disease risk.

However, they are also rich in carbs. You may be able to enjoy a small amount of them when you are on your keto diet, but make sure you know exactly how much you can eat before exceeding your carb limit.

Sugar

We mean sugar in any form, including honey. You may already be aware of what foods contain lots of sugar, such as cookies, candies, and cake are forbidden on a keto diet or any other form of diet that is designed to lose weight.

You may not be aware that nature's sugar, such as honey, is just as rich in carbs as processed sugar. Natural forms of sugar contain even more carbs.

Not only that sugar, in general, is rich in carbs, they also add little to no nutritional value to your meal. When you are on a keto diet, you need to keep in mind that your diet consists of food that is rich in fiber and nutritious. So, sugar is out of the question.

If you want to sweeten your food, you can use a healthy sweetener instead because they do not add as many carbs to your food.

Chips and Crackers

These two are some of the most popular snacks. What some people did not realize is that one packet of chips contains several servings and should not be all eaten in one go. The carbs can add up very quickly if you do not watch what you eat.

Crackers also pack a lot of carbs, although the amount varies based on how they are made. But even whole-wheat crackers contain a lot of carbs.

Due to how processed snacks are produced, it is difficult to stop eating everything within a short period. Therefore, it is advised that you avoid them altogether.

Milk

Milk contains a lot of carbs on its own. Therefore, avoid it if you can even though milk is a good source of many nutrients such as calcium, potassium, and other B vitamins.

Of course, that does not mean that you have to ditch milk altogether. You can get away with a tablespoon or two of milk for your coffee. But cream or half-and-half is better if you drink coffee frequently. These two contain very few carbs. But if you love to drink milk in large amounts or need it to make your favorite drinks, consider using coconut milk or unsweetened almond instead.

Gluten-free Baked Goods

Wheat, barley, and rye all contain gluten. Some people who have celiac disease still want to enjoy these delicacies but unable to because their gut will become inflamed in response to gluten. As such, gluten-free variants have been created to cater to their needs.

Gluten-free diets are very popular nowadays, but many people don't realize that they pack quite a lot of carbs. That includes gluten-free bread, muffins, and other baked products. In reality, they contain even more carbs than their glutenous variant. Moreover, the flour used to make these gluten-free products are made from grains and starches. So when you consume a gluten-free bread, your blood sugar level spikes.

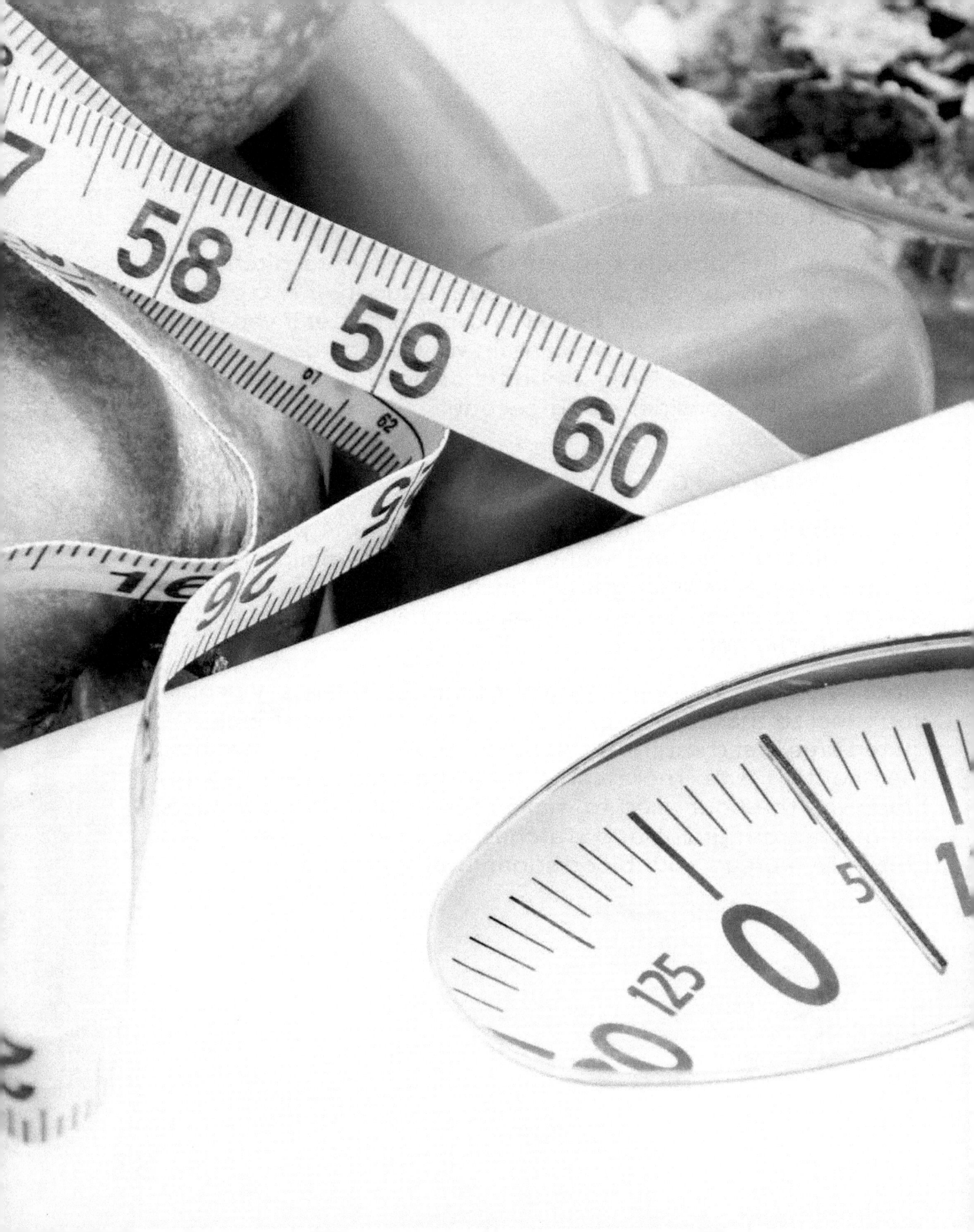

Chapter 04
Know Your Macros

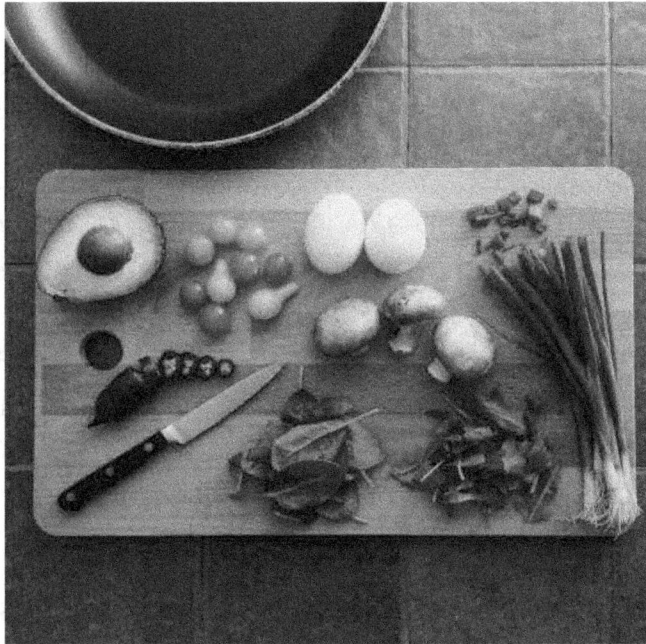

Every self-respecting diet must explain to the reader what macronutrients our body needs, how to calculate them, and how to manage them in the best possible way. There is no perfect diet; each of us is unique and different. We must learn to manage our diet completely independently. There are three macronutrients: carbohydrates, proteins, and fats.

Macronutrients are found in every food. They are the nutrients that fuel the body. Carbohydrates, proteins, and fats are included in the calories consumed and should be tracked while on the keto diet. The information needed is on the nutritional value label found on foods. Accurately measure individual portions to be sure to have accurate nutritional information. These nutrients being tracked are typically called "macros," a shortened version of the word macronutrient. By making adjustments to the SKD and HPKD, a gentler keto plan may be created to fit the needs of women over 50. First, we will look at the carbohydrates. You will be counting net carbs. Grams of net carbs are determined by subtracting the grams of dietary fiber and the grams of sugar alcohols from the grams of total carbohydrates. Dietary fiber does not release insulin into the body. The same is true of sugar alcohols. As a result, you will be able to eat more nutritionally, dense foods. You may satisfy your food cravings and hunger.

Next, we will look at fats. You will be eating 60 to 75% of your food as fat. This allows for a wide variety of foods, like bacon and pork rinds, to be included in your diet. Avocado, nuts, and other foods will be included in your diet as well. Because you will be eating food that is not processed, it will be important to eat healthy fats, including oil derived from natural food sources like avocado oil and coconut oil. High-quality butter and ghee will also be good sources of fat.

When we start to consider proteins, proteins do not need to be lean meats. The proteins included in Keto should not be lean but should be high in fat so that you consume appropriate amounts of fat. The keto diet is only effective when there is a high amount of fat consumed.

Now, let's start calculating the macros. To calculate the grams of net carbohydrates to include in your daily diet, it is important to determine your body weight and then your percentage of body fat. To do this, weigh yourself. After determining your weight, divide your body weight by your height in inches and square height in inches squared. Multiply that by 703, and you will have your BMI, or body mass index.

Lbs/height in inches, squared, times 703=BMI. So, in actuality, if you are a 5-foot 6-inch woman weighing 200 lbs. that's, $200/66^2$ x 703=32.28. The BMI is 32.28.

Then calculate your body fat percentage. (1.2 x BMI) + (.23 * age) - 5.4 equals body fat percentage. When we plug in the BMI from our female example, (1.2 * 32.28) + (.23*55) - 5.4 =45.98

So, the body fat percentage is 45.98%. Now that you have your body fat percentage, take your body fat percentage and multiply it by your body weight. 45.98% x 200 lb. That equals 91.96 lbs. of body fat. Subtract the body fat from your weight, and you have your LBM (Lean Body Mass). So, 200 - 91.96 equals 108.04. The LBM is 108.04.

Now, it's time to determine the number of macronutrients to eat each day.

We can start with the calculation for protein. There are .8 grams per pound of lean body mass. In our example, .8* 108.04 equals 84 grams. This is equal to 346 calories because there are four calories in each gram of protein. In our example, 20% of the calories the daily calories will be from protein. Therefore, 346 calories/.20 equals 1730 calories per day.

The total calories are 1730 calories per day.

To determine the number of carbohydrates, let's look at the number of carbohydrates in a gentler keto. 10% of the daily calories will come from carbs. 10% of 1730 calories is 173 calories. If you divide 173 calories by 4 (there are four calories in each carbohydrate), you will have 43.25g of carbohydrates as your daily allowance.

The remaining calories for each day will be fat:

346 Calories, Protein 86.50g 20%

+173 Calories, Carbohydrate 43.25g 10%

519 Calories of Protein and Carbs

-1730 (Total Daily Calories)

1211 Calories, Fat 134.56g 70%

There are nine calories in each fat gram. 1,211 calories/9 calories = 134.56g of fat for each day, or 70% of your daily calorie intake.

These macros will change as your BMI and LBM change. Make sure you adjust your macros every four or five weeks while you're losing weight so that your macros are accurate. You will want to record what you are eating and review your success in weight loss. This will allow you to track how your body is reacting to food combinations. Each body is different. It is important to see how you feel when you are eating different foods and combinations of foods as your approach ketosis. Be sure you're eating whole grains and getting fiber through leafy green vegetables. You will also want to be very familiar with nutrition labels to ensure you're not consuming hidden carbohydrates without realizing you are doing so.

Chapter 05
Why to follow keto diet after 50

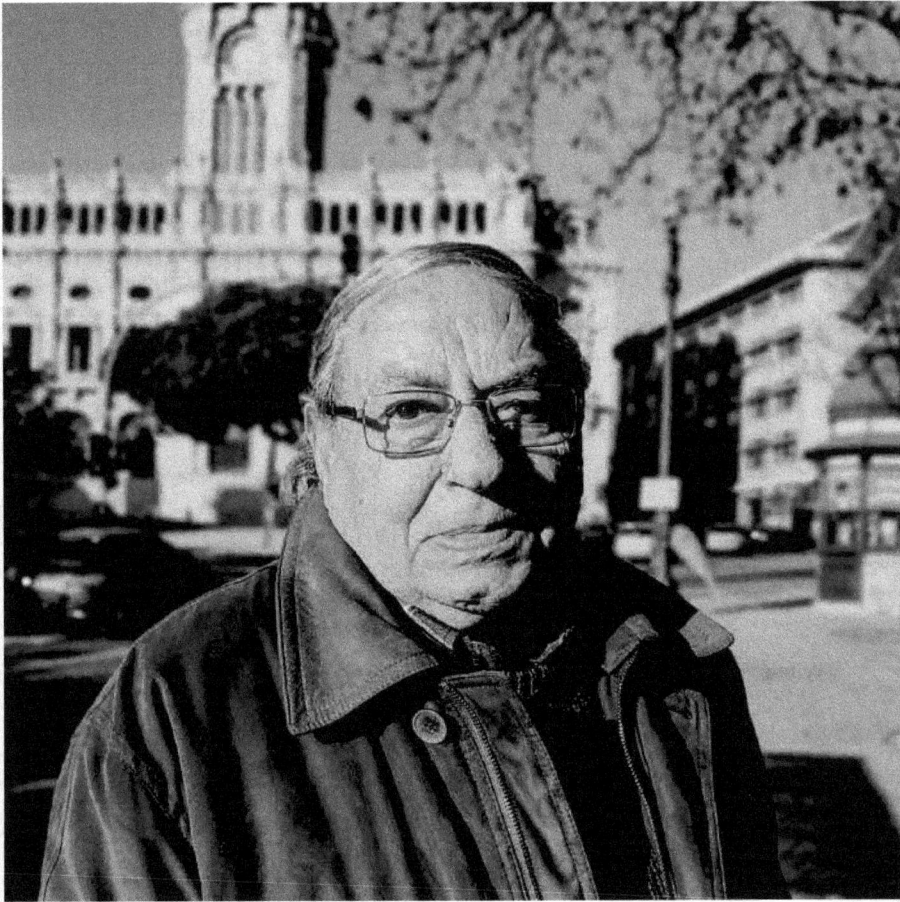

When you reach the age of 50, you will notice many changes in your body. Among the most common symptoms are a loss of muscle, the need for less sleep, and finer skin. You don't have to worry about this. Still, you have to pay much more attention than usual to your lifestyle. It is essential to keep fit, get exercise, and have a healthy and correct diet under all macros.

From this point of view, the ketogenic diet offers enormous advantages, as seen in the previous chapters. You can apply it even if you have health problems. Of course, a visit to a nutritionist can help you personalize your diet even more effectively. But this is "something more," the information in this book is more than enough, you just need to study it and apply it diligently.

As said, the functions of our body change according to age. The thing that changes most is our metabolism; it is physiological that it slows down with age. This change is due both to aging, but also to our lifestyle. Current metabolism is a consequence of our lifestyle in recent years.

A healthy lifestyle, with frequent, low-abundance meals, with moderate alcohol consumption, will have a faster metabolism than a lifestyle consisting of large meals eaten once a day, alcohol, and insomnia.

The ketogenic diet can help you from this point of view, eliminating carbohydrates and promoting the elimination of fats from our body. Another advantage is its flexibility; in fact, you can play with macros and adapt them to your needs, lifestyle, and progress made, of course.

Start gradually; your body has adapted for years to an unhealthy lifestyle, so do not overdo it overnight. Take your time and slowly reach your goals. There is no need to run; this is a marathon, not 100 meters.

At first, you may feel tired, tired, without energy. Don't worry; it's a normal thing; it's your body adapting to the new food style. You're taking away its main source of energy, carbohydrates; logically, it has to adapt. It must change the main energy source, it must switch to using fats, but this takes time, two or three days are necessary. The drop-in sugars could decrease your pressure for a couple of days, avoid exercise, and there will be no problems. The resulting benefits will be enormous.

KETO DIET FOR PEOPLE BELOW 50 VS KETO FOR ABOVE 50

Those who are younger than 50 years of age find that they can stick to traditional Keto diets with no problems. They have schedules, cheat days, and other tools that help them. Missing a day or two does not have too serious repercussions as they can make up. However, one over 50, Ketoing has to be taken more seriously simply because it is harder to lose weight.

Because it becomes harder to lose weight, many over 50's have made Ketoing the 'rule' and not the exception. This book's careful study will show that all the great recipes have been converted to Keto forms. Carbs were taken and replaced with fats, and proteins are highly favored.

When 50 or above, your Keto diet must be followed religiously. This used to be a problem as most of the things we loved just involved a lot of carbs. Luckily, that is no longer the case. With the right recipe book, you will find it much easier to do without carbs. Remember to run any dietary changes by your doctor.

KETO FOR WOMEN OVER 50

Women go through so much in life, don't we? From growing up, discovering the joys of life, pursuing a promising career, becoming a mother, there is so much that changes within such a short period.

While that is a part of life, what anyone would genuinely try and avoid would be where we put on excessive weight that we carry around like unneeded luggage. It is embarrassing, it is distracting, and it is causing quite a few internal issues.

If you thought the biggest hurdle you will face when you hit 50 is a big belly, think again. This isn't the only problem we face. While some would say that having a generous belly is the biggest problem, I firmly believe that there are more serious issues to worry about than that. When it comes to women, well, things aren't looking good.

Our bodies, since birth, continuously change. Most of these changes do not harm us and are only natural. However, once we enter into our 50s, things are a lot different. Now, any changes within our body will directly affect how we perform, operate, and work. If we were to keep these changes unchecked and pay no close attention, things would take a worse turn.

Most of these issues will remain the same for men; however, due to the chemistry of our bodies and differences, both internal and external, both would face a variety of issues exclusive to their gender.

There are a few ways we can avoid these issues. Some of these ways require you to go back in time and start working out from a very young age, control your diet, and change your habits. That is the stuff of science fiction and hence is out of the equation.

Other ways would include visiting a doctor and getting pills and energy boosters to help us feel better while taking more pills to fight diabetes, high blood pressure, and other health issues. This way is not just hectic but far too complicated as well.

For a very long time, the only other way was to avoid worrying too much and hope that life would fix issues itself, and that never ended well for many. People have then left with worry and a gap that nothing was able to fill. In comes ketogenic diet.

Call it a need of the hour, a savior in disguise, or anything you like. The fact remains that this is proving to be a popular option that is not only delivering results but is also helping millions to maintain a healthy lifestyle and reverse some of the damage their bodies have suffered.

Numerous studies have supported the idea that keto diets are far more effective for older men and women than the younger folks. With so much to look forward to and so little to sacrifice, it does make sense to state that Keto is essentially becoming your permanent way of life once you hit 50, but why is that? Why do I and so many others proclaim Keto as an important lifestyle choice for women above 50? The answer to this involves some explanation, but I will do my best to do just that!

As a woman, you have likely experienced significant differences in the way you must diet compared to how men can diet. Women tend to have a harder time losing weight because of their different hormones and how their bodies break down fats. Another factor to consider is your age group. As the body ages, it is important to be more attentive with the way that you care for yourself. Aging bodies start to experience problems more quickly, and this can be avoided with the proper diet and exercise plan. Keto works well for women of all ages, and this is because of how it communicates with the body. No matter how fit you are right now or how much weight you need or want to lose, Keto will change the way that your body metabolizes, giving you a very personalized experience.

When starting your Keto diet, you should not be thinking about extremes because that isn't what Keto should be about. You should be able to place your body into ketosis without feeling terrible in the process. One of the biggest guidelines to follow while starting your Keto journey is to regularly listen to your body. If you ever feel that you are starving or simply unfulfilled, then you will likely have to modify the way you are eating because it isn't reaching ketosis properly. It is not an overnight journey, so you need to remember to be patient with yourself and with your body. Adapting to a Keto diet takes a bit of transition time and a lot of awareness.

The health benefits of the Keto diet are not different for men or women, but the speed at which they are reached does differ. As mentioned, women's bodies are a lot different when it comes to how they can burn fats and lose weight. For example, by design, women have at least 10% more body fat than men. No matter how fit you are, this is just an aspect of being a woman that you must consider. Don't be hard on yourself if you notice that it seems like men can lose weight easier — that's because they can! What women have in additional body fat, men typically have the same in muscle mass. This is why men tend to see faster external results. That added muscle mass means that their metabolism rates are higher. That increased metabolism means that fat and energy get burned faster. When you are on Keto, though, the internal change is happening right away.

Your metabolism is unique, but it is also going to be slower than a man's by nature. Since muscle can burn more calories than fat, the weight just seems to fall off men, giving them the ability to quickly reach the opportunity for muscle growth. This should not be something that holds you back from starting your Keto journey. As long as you keep these realistic bodily factors in mind, you won't be left wondering why it is taking you a little longer to start losing weight. This point will come for you, but it will take a bit more of a process you must be committed to following through with.

Another unique condition that a woman can experience, but a man cannot be PCOS or Polycystic Ovary Syndrome; a hormonal imbalance that causes cysts' development. These cysts can cause pain, interfere with normal reproductive function, and, in extreme and dangerous cases, burst. PCOS is very common among women, affecting up to 10% of the entire female population. Surprisingly, most women are not even aware that they have the condition. Around 70% of women have PCOS, which is undiagnosed. This condition can cause a significant hormonal imbalance, therefore affecting your metabolism. It can also inevitably lead to weight gain, making it even harder to see results while following diet plans. To stay on top of your health, you must make sure that you are going to the gynecologist regularly.

Menopause is another reality that must be faced by women, especially as we age. Most women begin the process of menopause in their mid-40s. Men do not go through menopause, so they are spared from yet another condition that causes slower metabolism and weight gain. When you start menopause, it is easy to gain weight and lose muscle. Once menopause begins, most women lose muscle at a much faster rate and conversely gain weight, despite dieting and exercise regimens. Keto can, therefore, be the right diet plan for you. Regardless of what your body is doing naturally, via processes like menopause, your internal systems are still going to be making the switch from running on carbs to deriving energy from fats.

When the body begins to run on fats successfully, you have an automatic fuel reserve waiting to be burned. It will take some time for your body to do this. However, when it does, you will be able to eat fewer calories and still feel full because your body knows to take energy from the fat you already have. This will become automatic. However, it is a process that requires some patience, but being aware of what is going on with your body can help you stay motivated while on Keto.

Because a Keto diet reduces the amount of sugar you are consuming, it naturally lowers insulin in your bloodstream. This can have amazing effects on any existing PCOS and fertility issues and menopausal symptoms and conditions like pre-diabetes and Type 2 diabetes. Once your body adjusts to a Keto diet, you are overcoming the things that are naturally in place that can be preventing you from losing weight and getting healthy. Even if you placed your body on a strict diet, if it isn't getting rid of sugars properly, you likely aren't going to see the same results that you will when you try Keto. This is a big reason why Keto can be so beneficial for women.

For women over 50, there are guidelines to follow when you start your Keto diet. As long as you follow the method properly and listen to what your body truly needs, you should have no more problems than men do while following the plan. What you will have are more obstacles to overcome, but you can do it. Remember that plenty of women successfully follow a Keto diet and see great results. Use these women as inspiration for how you anticipate your journey to go. When it seems impossible, remember what you have working against you, but more importantly, what you have working for you. Your body is designed to go into ketogenesis more than it is designed to store fat by overeating carbs. Use this as a motivation to keep pushing you ahead. Keto is a valid option for you, and the results will prove this, especially if you are over the age of 50.

There comes an age in a woman's life where her menstrual cycle will finally end. This is a phrase that means your ovaries stop releasing eggs, better known as ovulation, and therefore menstruation ends. This condition is generally observed in women above the age of 40. No defined age shows when a woman can expect menopause.

There are times where women may experience menopause prematurely as well. This happens if a woman has undergone surgeries like hysterectomy (surgery that involves the removal of ovaries). It can also happen from any injuries that may have caused damage to the ovaries. If this happens before the age of 40, it is classified as premature menopause.

Menopause, as harmless as it sounds, can be quite a troubling phase for women. The hot flashes you experience will keep you up at night, with an elevated heartbeat. The constant feeling of being irritated and a clear downfall in your sex life can contribute greatly towards you feeling more and more grumpy.

Menopause takes a toll on your hormonal balance. The newly developed imbalance then pushes your body to gain massive weight, experience mood swings like never before, and a libido that is crashing faster than you can imagine.

KETO FOR MEN OVER 50

Men also go through quite a lot of internal and external changes. These include but are not limited to physical changes, habitual changes, and so on. While the chemistry inside the body of both remains broadly the same, whether young or old, there are things which men are more likely to develop or lose than women, these include some diseases, ailments, infections, frequent changes, and disorders. The worst news is, it happens as soon as you cross 45 years of age. That means you are at least five years late already, or that is what you think.

KETO FOR WOMEN VS. MEN

In reality, since women and men have been created differently, our approach to Keto Diet may differ and should be different. These are the biological indifferences that we have no control with. We will be discussing the differences between males and females when it comes to approaching the Keto Diet.

So how should men do it or women do it? Here's a thing we need to understand about the Keto Diet. First and foremost is that it is a very bio-individual. Even among men, there are different ways to do it. Among women, there are different ways, as well. Just understand that it is individual, and it might take some tweaking as you go throughout the process. But for all men and all women, it's really important to become Keto adaptive first before we start tweaking things, so what we mean by that is you need to do Keto strict for the first thirty days or so until you get adapted. Your body is becoming more efficient, and it is adapting to this new fuel source called ketones. It is going to take a while before your body gets adapted. But once you get adapted here, there might be some difference in men versus women, so some women tend not to do well over the long term with intermittent fasting.

So, a lot of people that do Keto do intermittent fasting as well because it puts you in a modified or a modified state of ketosis, so you are making some ketones but women over the long term because of their hormones being different with men and their cycles during that time of the month. They might need to increase their carbohydrate intakes the week before their cycle starts.

So what we recommend to all women out there is that if you have become adapted to the Ketogenic Diet is that you should be cycling in and out of ketosis from time to time and specifically try it out adding in healthy carbs, not pizza, French fries or soda but healthy carbs like fruit, potatoes, sweet potatoes, maybe a little bit of rice the week before your cycle. Adding those carbohydrates during nighttime could help balance those hormones so that you don't experience their side effects from going Keto long term. And that is what we've seen help a lot of women that are clients is adding those in plus you are not as grumpy or angry. This stuff can help out with those symptoms and side effects. So, add in carbohydrates the week before your cycle.

For men also, it is best recommended that you test your hormones and get your blood work done every couple of months, so you know how your body is changing and adapting so you know maybe you need to switch things up or maybe do the target a ketogenic diet for a week or two and see how your body responds and adapts. You need to become your experimentations, so you know what is best for you moving forward.

The truth is, there is a wide variety of people who can benefit from the Ketogenic Diet, whether they are young, old, man, or woman. Still, the Ketogenic Diet has been especially beneficial for women due to their different hormones and conditions.

HOW TO START A KETO DIET WHEN YOU'RE OVER 50?

Once you have made your decision, the next thing to do is speak to your doctor about it. As discussed, whether or not you're suffering from a medical condition, it's important to speak to your doctor to learn more about the keto diet and if it's right for you. Let's take a look at some steps to take when getting started:

Do Your Research on Keto-friendly Food

First of all, you need to acquire a list of foods to eat and avoid. Depending on your budget and location, some of those foods may be difficult to find. So you may want to look for food alternatives that are also keto-friendly. Also, learn how to spot "hidden carbs" in the food items you purchase. Many foods may claim to be keto-friendly but may contain additional carbs or sugars.

Practice Portion Control

Just because you're allowed to eat foods rich in fats and proteins, doesn't mean you should eat excessive amounts. Although you don't have to count calories every time you eat, you should practice portion control so you don't go overboard. This is where a high-quality food scale comes in handy.

Be Prepared to Experience Some Side Effects

Although these side effects don't happen to most people, you might be unlucky enough to experience them. One of the most common side effects is a condition known as the "keto flu." You will know that you have this condition if you experience side effects such as headaches, fatigue, irritability, a lack of motivation, brain fog (an inability to focus), sugar cravings, muscle cramps, dizziness, and nausea. However, if you already know what to watch out for, you don't have to worry. Most of these side effects are temporary and will go away. Also, try not to let the side effects discourage you from sticking with the diet.

Exercise

This is optional, but you should take care of your muscles at your age as they start to degrade. You will feel better, your health will improve, and your weight will go down faster.

Consult a Nutrition Specialist

This book is a valuable tool to get an idea of what a ketogenic diet is, what the benefits are, and how to avoid classic mistakes. It is a complete guide, with which, if studied well, you will certainly be able to set your diet according to your daily needs. However, consulting a doctor is never a bad idea; you can discuss your opinions and give you valuable advice. I recommend consulting your doctor, especially in cases of health problems and cases where you have never been on a diet.

Chapter 06

Keto Benefits, Not Only Weight Loss

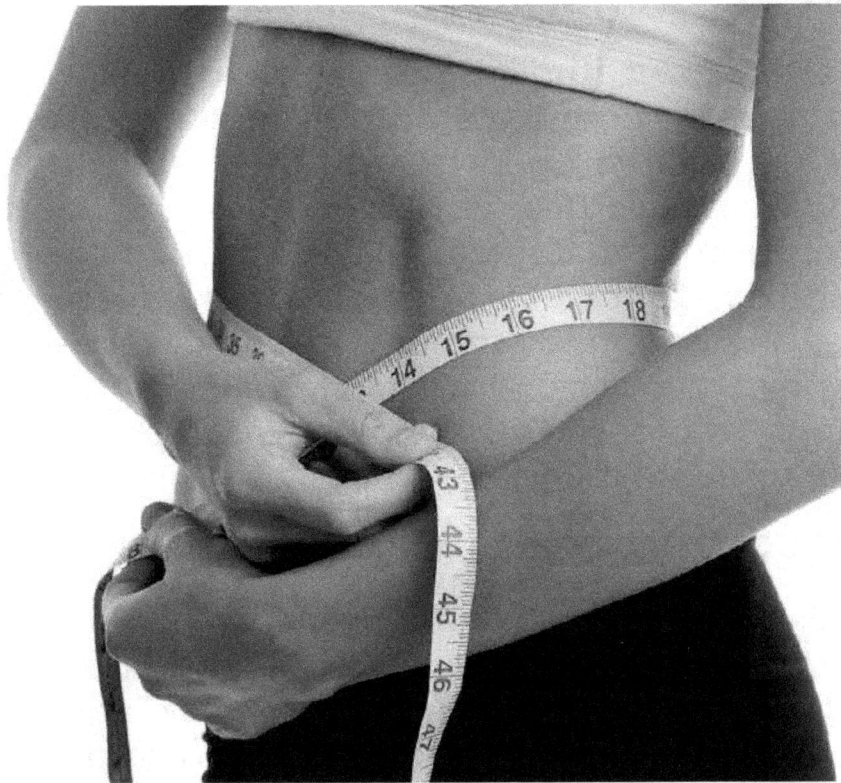

The Keto diet has been proven to have many advantages for people over 50. Here are some of the best.

STRENGTHENS BONES

When people get older, their bones weaken. At 50, your bones at likely not as strong as they used to be; however, you can keep them in really good conditions. Consuming milk to give calcium cannot do enough to strengthen your bones. What you can do is make use of the Keto diet as it is low in toxins. Toxins negatively affect the absorption of nutrients, and so with this, your bones can take in all they need.

IT ERADICATES NUTRIENTS DEFICIENCY

Keto focuses on consuming exactly what you need. If you use a great Keto plan, your body will lack no nutrients and will not suffer any deficiency.

REDUCED HUNGER

The reason we find it hard to stick to diets is hunger. It doesn't matter your age; diets do not become easier to stick to. We may have a mental picture of the healthy body we want. We may even have clear visuals of the kind of life we want to leave once free from unhealthy living, but none of that matters when hunger enters the scene. However, the Keto diet is a diet that combats this problem. Keto diet focuses on consuming plenty of proteins. Proteins are filling and do not let you feel hungry too easily. Also, when your carb levels are reduced, your appetite takes a hit. It is a win-win situation.

REDUCES BLOOD SUGAR AND INSULIN

After 50, monitoring blood sugar can be a real struggle. Cutting down on cars drastically reduces both insulin levels and blood sugar levels. This means that the Keto diet will benefit millions as many people struggle with insulin complications and high blood sugar levels. It has been proven to help as when some people embark on Keto, they cut up to half of the carbs they consume. It's a treasure for those with diabetes and insulin resistance. A study was carried out on people with type 2 diabetes.

INCREASES HDL LEVELS

HDL refers to high-density lipoprotein. When your HDL levels are compared to your LDL levels and are not found low, your risk of developing heart disease is lowered. This is great for persons over 50 as heart diseases suddenly become more probable. Eating fats and reducing carbohydrates intake is one of the most assured ways to increase your high-density lipoprotein levels.

BRAIN BENEFITS

As you begin to change the fuel source for your body, this includes significant fuel sources for your brain. Studies have found that individuals were able to increase the stability of their neurons through the Ketogenic Diet as well as the up-regulation of the mitochondrial enzymes and brain mitochondria.

IMPROVED ENDURANCE AND MUSCLE GAIN

As we get older, we generally begin to lose the muscle mass we once had. As mentioned earlier, one of the main ketones you will begin producing as you begin the Ketogenic Diet is BHB. BHB helps promote muscle gain. When you combine the ketogenic diet with proper exercise, you will be increasing your health and muscle gain at the same time.

IMPROVE SLEEP AND ENERGY LEVELS

Unfortunately, many individuals underestimate how important sleep is. The good news is that after only four or five days on the ketogenic diet, many individuals have reported that they already begin to benefit from higher energy levels. On a scientific level, this may be because, through your new ketogenic diet, you will be stabilizing your insulin levels. As your body becomes stabilized, this will help provide you with a ready energy source rather than experiencing the spikes and crashes.

WEIGHT LOSS

Weight loss is one of the major reasons anyone begins a diet. Luckily through the ketogenic diet, there is substantial evidence that by eating the proper foods, you will be able to lose weight and preserve your muscle mass. In a related study, it was found that individuals who followed a ketogenic diet, compared to individuals on a low-calorie and low-fat diet, were able to lose weight at 2.2 times! These people also improved their HDL cholesterol and Triglyceride levels.

BONE HEALTH

Osteoporosis becomes more likely as a person advances in age. This is especially true if you weren't able to introduce appropriate amounts of calcium in your body. As you probably know, osteoporosis makes the bone brittle and fragile. This means that your likelihood of having a serious injury from seemingly small accidents increases. A simple slip and bones can fracture, or hips may become dislocated.

INCREASED METABOLIC HEALTH

An important factor behind these issues is insulin. Insulin plays a vital role as far as metabolic disease and diabetes go. Luckily, the Ketogenic Diet is very effective in lowering insulin levels for individuals who are prediabetic or have type 2 diabetes.

IMPROVES IMMUNE SYSTEM

While healthy cells can easily switch to burning ketones for energy, cancer cells are not that lucky, which means they grow significantly more slowly than they otherwise would when deprived of their primary food source. Switching to the keto diet is also ideal when it comes to promoting brain health for several reasons. The most important of these is that following the keto diet is closer to the way early humans likely ate, which means it is more in line with the type of fuel that the brain is naturally used to consuming.

MAY LOWER BLOOD PRESSURE

High blood pressure plagues adults much more than it does young ones. Once you attain 50, you must monitor your blood pressure rates. Reduction in the intake of carbohydrates is a proven way to lower your blood pressure. When you cut down on your carbs and lower your blood sugar levels, you greatly reduce your chances of getting some other diseases.

INCREASE LIFESPAN

During the ketogenic diet, insulin levels decrease. This will allow your body to use ketones for energy. Lowering oxidative stress and insulin level helps to increase your lifespan. One of the research studies proves that at the time of starvation, our body produces a chemical compound known as hydroxybutyrate. It plays an important role in the process of aging. Daily calorie restrictions are slow down the aging process and increase your lifespan.

REGULATE BLOOD SUGAR

Keto diet helps regulate blood sugar by controlling how much insulin is in the system. Maintaining the right insulin level is important because you can avoid problems such as insulin resistance or pre-diabetes. Keto diet has also been shown to reduce HbA1c levels, a measure of blood glucose control.

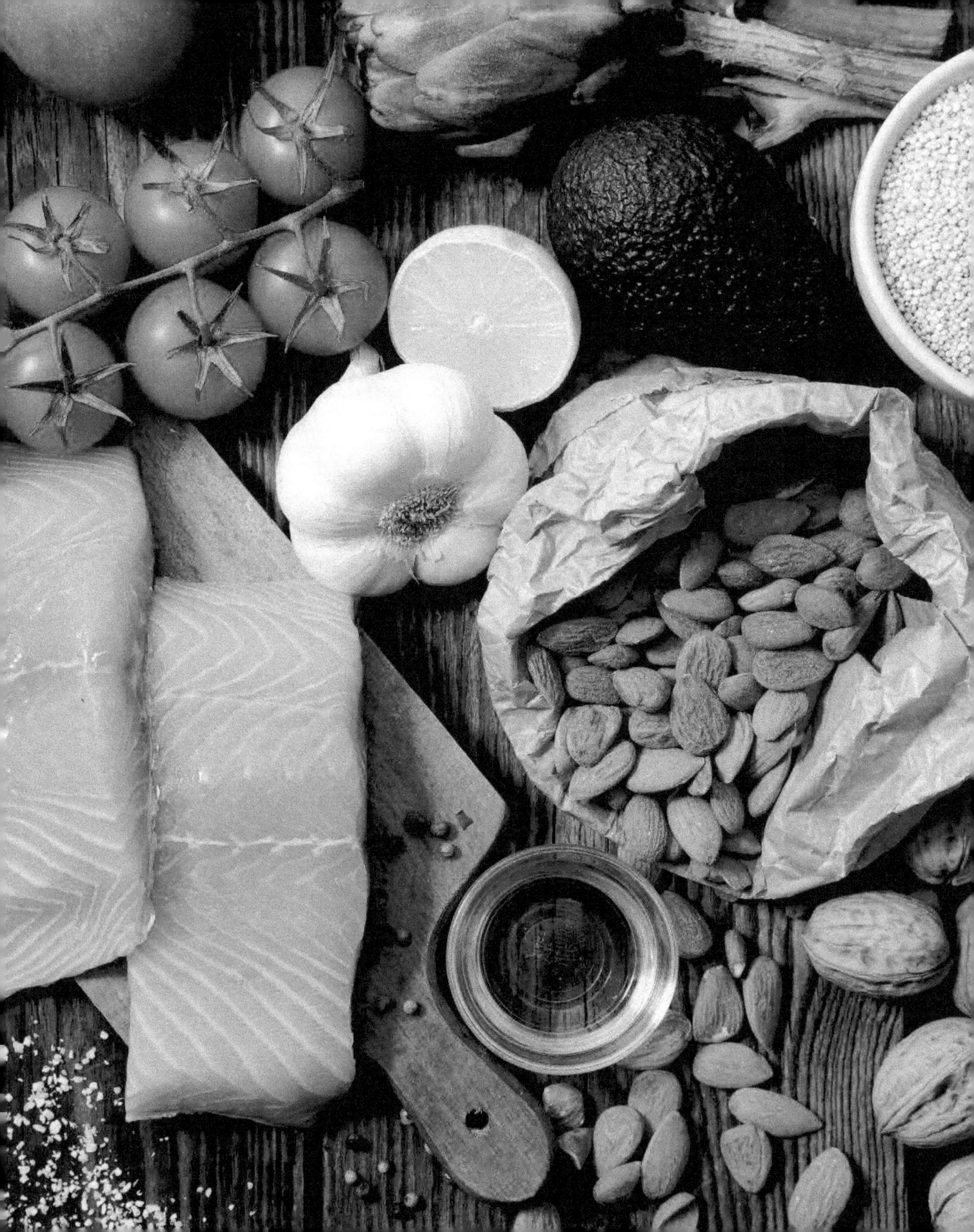

Chapter 07

Overcome Common Hurdles

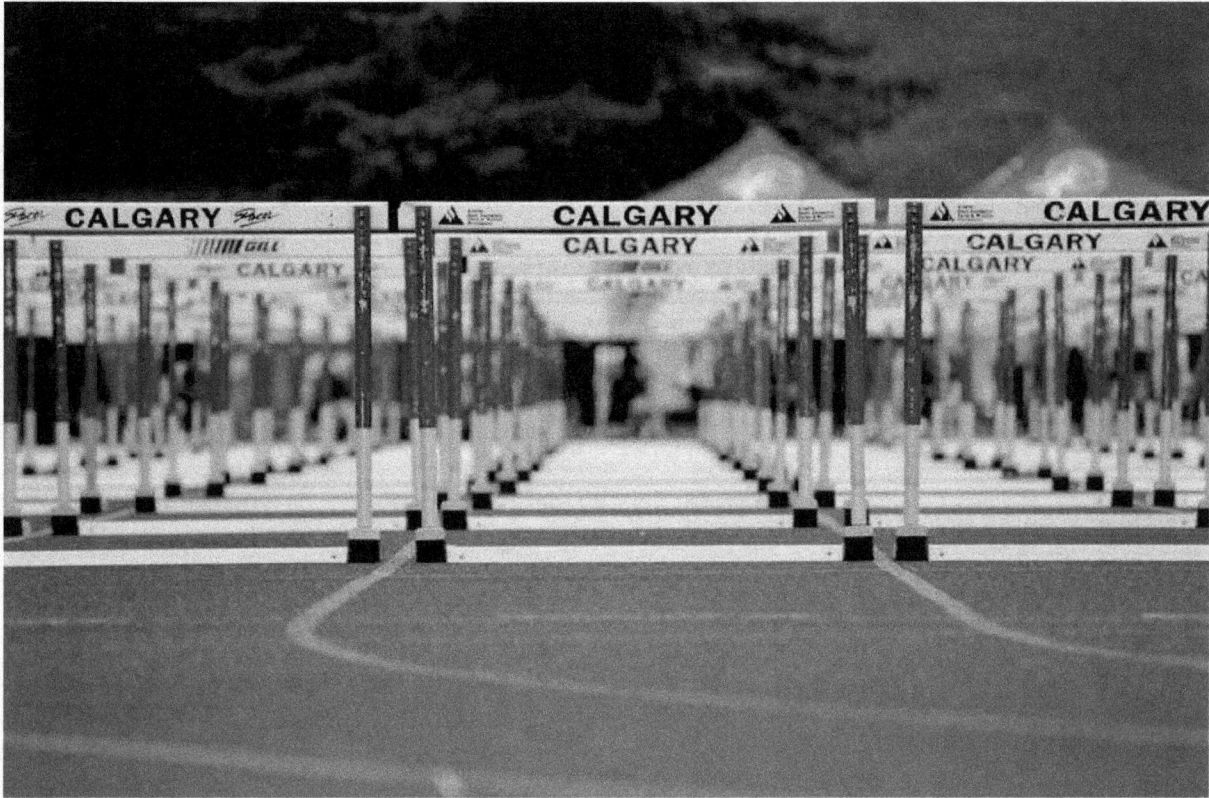

All types of diet can have negative effects because your body has gotten used to bad habits. Once you make the shift to a more positive way of eating, the body sort of goes on a rebellious phase, so it feels like everything is going wrong. For example, a person who used to eat lots of sugar in a day can have severe headaches once they start to avoid sugar. This is a withdrawal symptom and tells you that your diet is making positive changes to the body – albeit it takes a little bit of pain on your part.

So, what can one expect when they make that change towards a healthy Ketogenic Diet? Here are some of the things to expect and, of course – how to troubleshoot these problems.

KETO FLU

The Keto Flu is the most prominent problem you'll encounter when starting the diet. It's a perfectly normal reaction by the body that may seem alarming because, well, the symptoms don't feel good. You have to understand; your body has been running on a specific type of gasoline for years. It's been taking fuel from sugar, and with the Ketogenic Diet, it's like you're changing your fuel source to a cleaner and more sustainable type. It makes sense that the engine growls a little in protest – but after that, you'll be able to run beautifully without the guilt.

The Keto Flu has the following symptoms:

- Headaches
- Fatigue
- Irritability
- Brain fog or difficulty focusing
- Motivational problems
- Sugar cravings
- Dizziness
- Nausea
- Muscle cramps

FREQUENT URINATION

These symptoms are all heavily dependent on the kind of person doing the Keto Diet. Since you're already in our 50s, the symptoms may be more prominent, especially if you rely heavily on carbohydrates in your diet. If you eat mostly low-carb food, however, these effects may not be as obvious.

But how do you solve them? Here are some of the best ways to get rid of the Keto Flu as quickly as possible!

First, increase your water and salt consumption. This happens a lot once you start a Ketogenic Diet. You may not notice it, but a lot of the salt you consume is through carbohydrates like bread, pasta, rice, and so on. Salt tends to make you thirsty, so if you eat little salt, you're also less likely to look for water during the day. So, what happens now? Every time you feel dizzy or tired or nauseous while on a Keto Diet, just dissolve salt in water and gulp it down. This is not going to taste good - but I promise that it will help you feel better. You can always try consuming the salt and water separately – whatever you find most convenient. As for water, try to hit a target of 3 liters of water every day. The good news is that this doesn't have to be plain water – your smoothies, coffee, and tea drinks are also counted.

Add more fat to your diet. Because of all the wrong information circulating today, a lot of people are afraid of fat. We've discussed this before, but it bears repeating – fat is not your enemy. During the Ketogenic Diet, it makes sense to eat lots of fats, especially if your carbohydrate intake dips to an all-time low. If you lower the carbohydrate consumption without an equal fat increase, you will always feel hungry and tired.

Don't be impatient – go slower. Remember what we said about the body changing fuels when you're switching to the Ketogenic Diet? Well, the changing process doesn't have to be overnight. Choose to convert one meal at a time to a Keto-friendly set instead of changing all of them on your first day. Of course, it's recommended that you only do this if the saltwater method doesn't. Just remember – the Keto Flu will pass, so the first few days of discomfort should not discourage you. If you want to minimize the trouble, try starting your Ketogenic Diet on a low-stress period – like a holiday. So basically, instead of eating less than 50 grams of carbohydrates a day, you can have a target of 50 to 70.

Do NOT count calories or restrict your food consumption. When it comes to the Ketogenic Diet – you don't have to calorie count. Again, you don't want to stuff yourself with food because you don't have to count calories. The truth is that calories do not matter so much when your body is at a state of ketosis. It doesn't matter how many you're getting – your body will always break down the fat deposits, and there will be weight loss. Stressing about the calorie intake or depriving yourself of food because of the calories can worsen Keto Flu symptoms and make it more difficult for you to stick to the diet. The bottom line is this: as long as you're eating the allowed food items in allowed portions, you're OK.

Limit your physical activity. That's the good news with the Ketogenic Diet – you don't have to exercise. Sure, you may not be running marathons or going to the gym every week, but if you're health-conscious, then chances are you do light walks on a routine basis. That's perfectly OK – as long as you don't over-exert yourself. Now, there will be days when you will feel too good. Like you can go out and exercise because you have all this extra energy. When this happens, resist the temptation to do too much too soon. Your body is already burning as much fat as it can – don't push it too hard or get sick. If you're restless, try doing yoga, light walking, or just stretching.

Take some supplements. People using the Ketogenic Diet for a long time may also have vitamin and mineral deficiencies. It's not easily obvious, but it could happen, so you'll have to be prepared. The usual vitamins and minerals lacking in a Ketogenic Diet include calcium, zinc, selenium, and vitamin D – so try taking a multivitamin during your diet. Again, I can't stress this enough: always consult your doctor before taking any medication. This is especially true if you have pre-existing health problems and are also taking medication for maintenance.

CONSTIPATION OR DIARRHEA

These problems are fairly common because, well, you're changing your diet! Your body will react one way or another. In both cases, the solution is practically the same – water and fiber. Make sure you get enough fluids in your system and take fiber supplements through many stores. You can also try taking laxatives that are made, especially without carbohydrates.

If alarming symptoms occur while you're on the Ketogenic Diet, I want you to consult your doctor ASAP! Again, reactions may vary from one person to the next, and I don't want you shrugging off certain symptoms as if they're just "part" of the diet. Stay motivated, but also be mindful of what is happening to your body. Remember – we want you to be healthy!

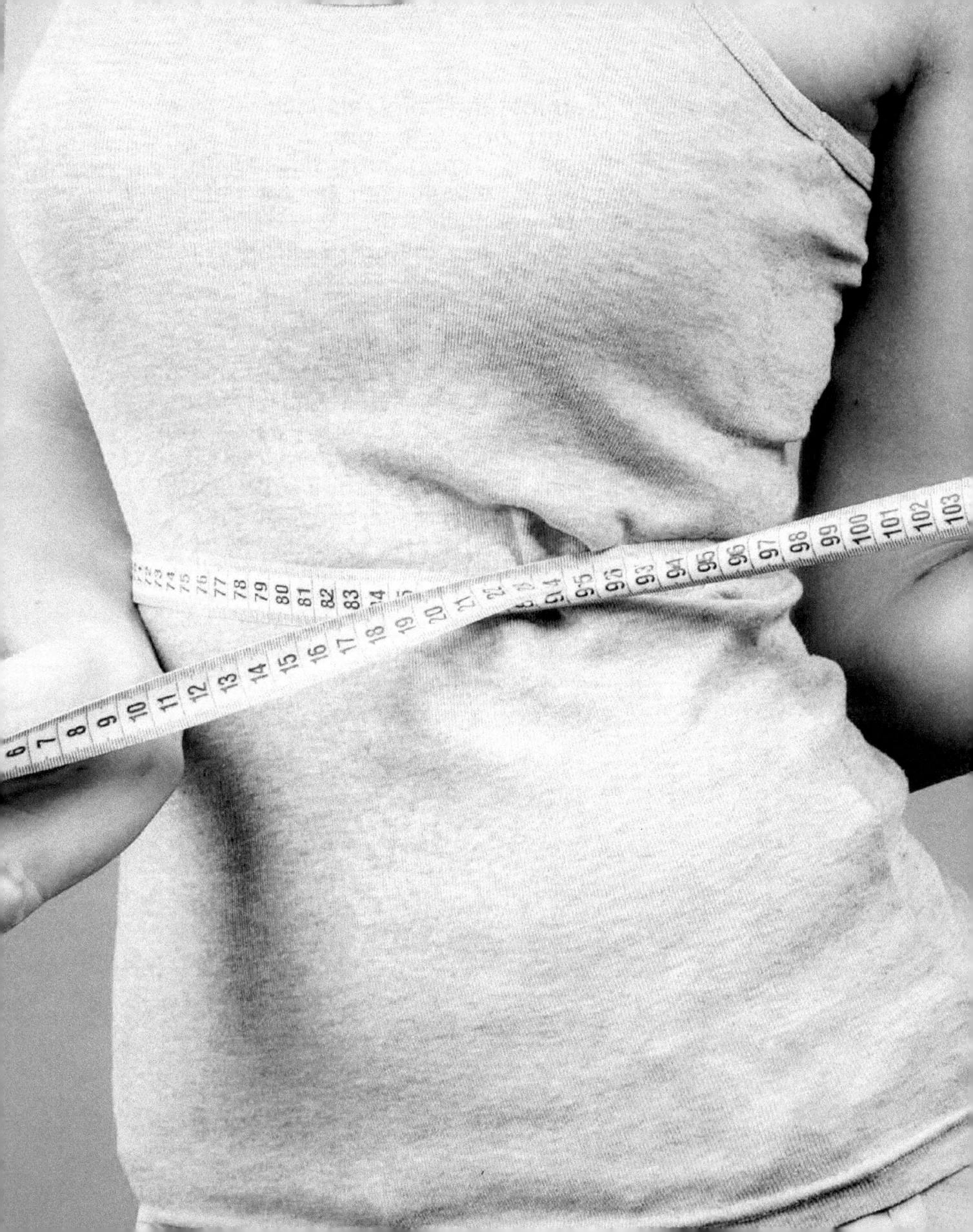

Chapter 08

Tips for Seniors Who Want to Start, That You will Not Find Elsewhere

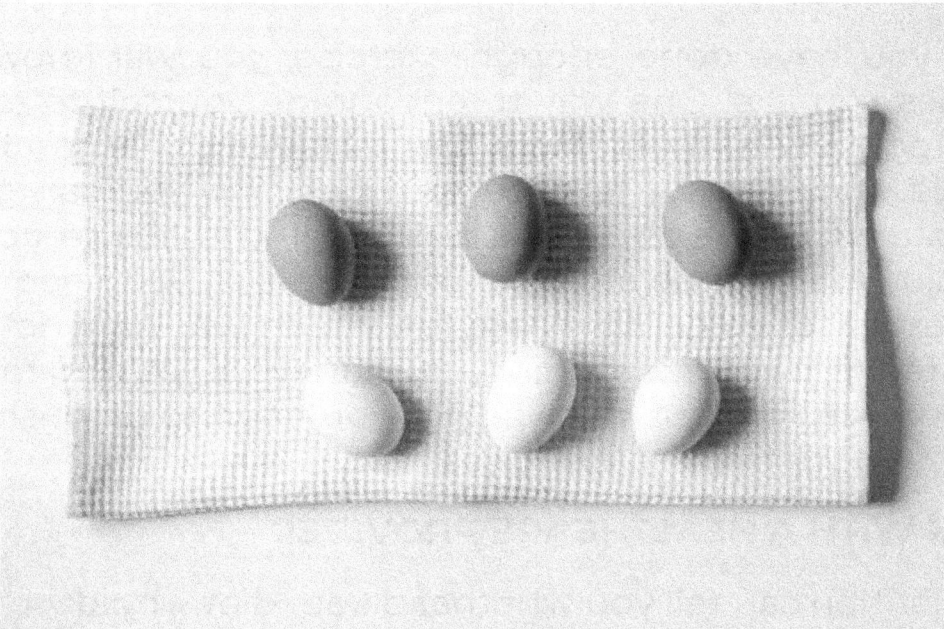

LEARN HOW TO COUNT YOUR MACROS

This is especially important at the start of your journey. As time goes by, you will learn how to estimate your meals without using a food scale.

PREPARE YOUR KITCHEN FOR YOUR KETO-FRIENDLY FOODS

Once you've made a choice, it's time to get rid of all the foods in your kitchen that aren't allowed in the keto diet. To do this, check the nutritional labels of all the food items. Of course, there's no need to throw everything away. You can donate foods you don't need to food kitchens and other institutions that give food to the needy.

PURCHASE SOME KETO STRIPS FOR YOURSELF

These are important so you can check your ketone levels and track your progress. You can purchase keto strips in pharmacies and online. For instance, some of the best keto strips available on Amazon are Perfect Keto Ketone Test Strips, Smackfat Ketone Strips, and One Earth Ketone Strips.

FIND AN ACTIVITY YOU ENJOY

When you have done enough exercise, you will know what activities you like. One way to encourage yourself to exercise more regularly is by making it entertaining than a chore. If possible, stick to your favorite activities, and you can get the most out of your exercises. Keep in mind that the activities you enjoy may not be effective or needed, so you need to find other exercises to compensate for, which you may not enjoy. For instance, if you like jogging, you can work your leg muscles, but your arms are not involved. So, you need to do pushups or other strength training exercises.

CHECK WITH A HEALTHCARE PROVIDER

Your dietitian can tell you whether a keto diet would work. Still, it helps to check in with your healthcare provider to ensure that you do not have any medical condition that prevents you from losing weight, such as hypothyroidism and polycystic ovarian syndrome. It helps to know well in advance whether your body is even capable of losing fat in the first place before you commit and see no result, right?

HYDRATE PROPERLY

That means drinking enough water or herbal tea and ditch sweetened beverages or other drinks that contain sugar altogether. Making the transition will be difficult for the first few weeks, but your body will be thanking you for it. There is nothing healthier than good old plain water, and the recommended amount is 2 gallons a day.

SUPPLEMENTS

When you get older, your body starts to lose its ability to absorb certain nutrients, which leads to deficits. For example, vitamin B12 and folate are some of the most common nutrients that people over 50 lack. They have an impact on your mood, energy level, and weight loss rate.

HAVE THE RIGHT MINDSET

Your mindset is one of the most important things you need to change when you've decided to follow the keto lifestyle. Without the right mindset, you might not stick with the diet long enough to enjoy all its benefits. Also, the proper mindset will keep you motivated to keep going no matter what challenges come your way.

GET ENOUGH SLEEP

Getting enough sleep helps your body regulate the hormones in your body, so try to aim for 7 to 9 hours of sleep a day. You can get more restful sleep by creating a nighttime routine that involves not looking at a computer, phone, or TV screen for at least 1 hour before bed. You can drink warm milk or water to help your body relax or even do 10 to 20 minutes of stretching to get a restful sleep.

KEEP A FOOD LOG

Then add the calories and divide by three to get an average. Now that you know how many takes, you can figure out how much you need to pay on average per day to reach your goals.

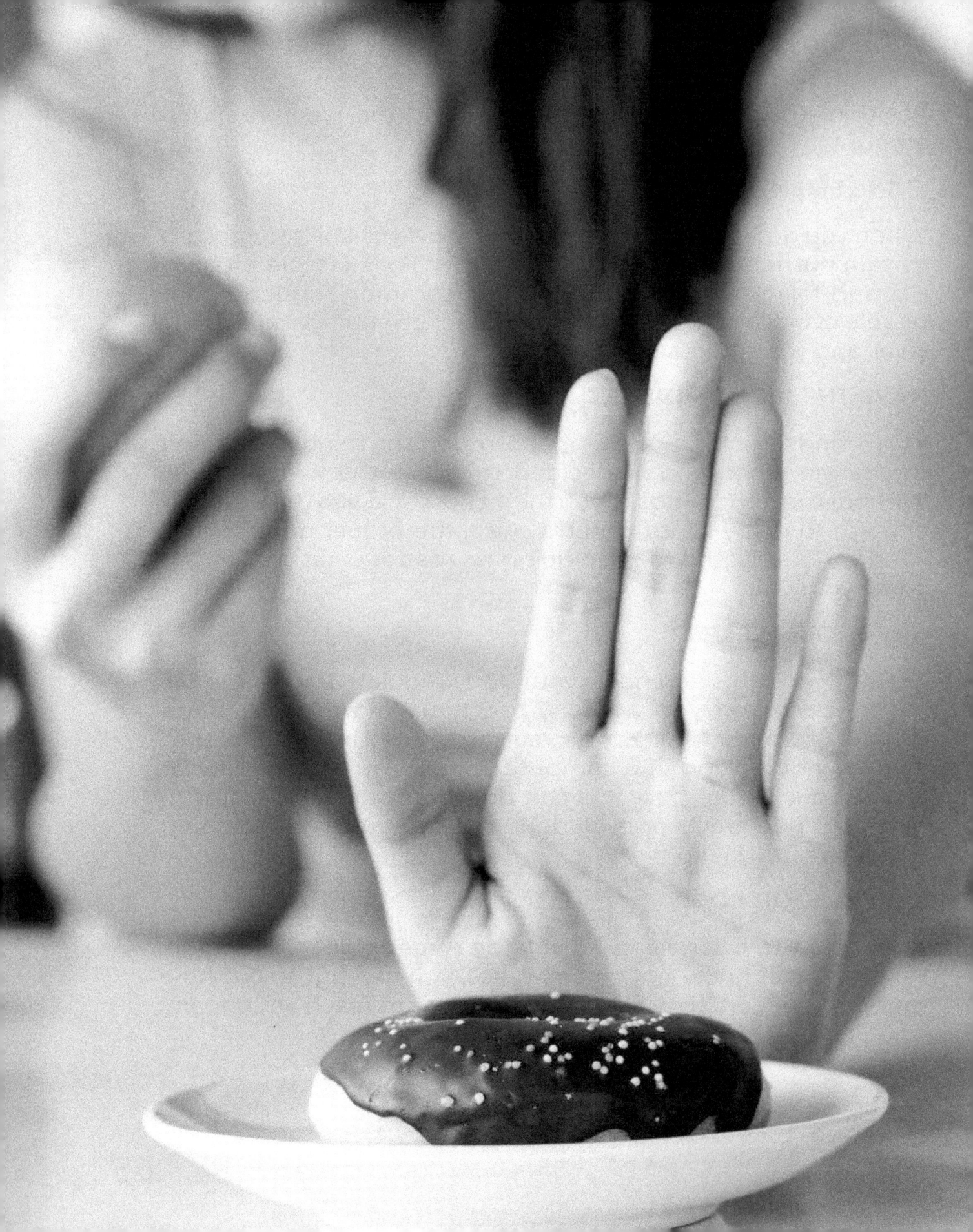

Chapter 09

The Ultimate Keto Shopping List for Saving Money and Time Without Wasting Food

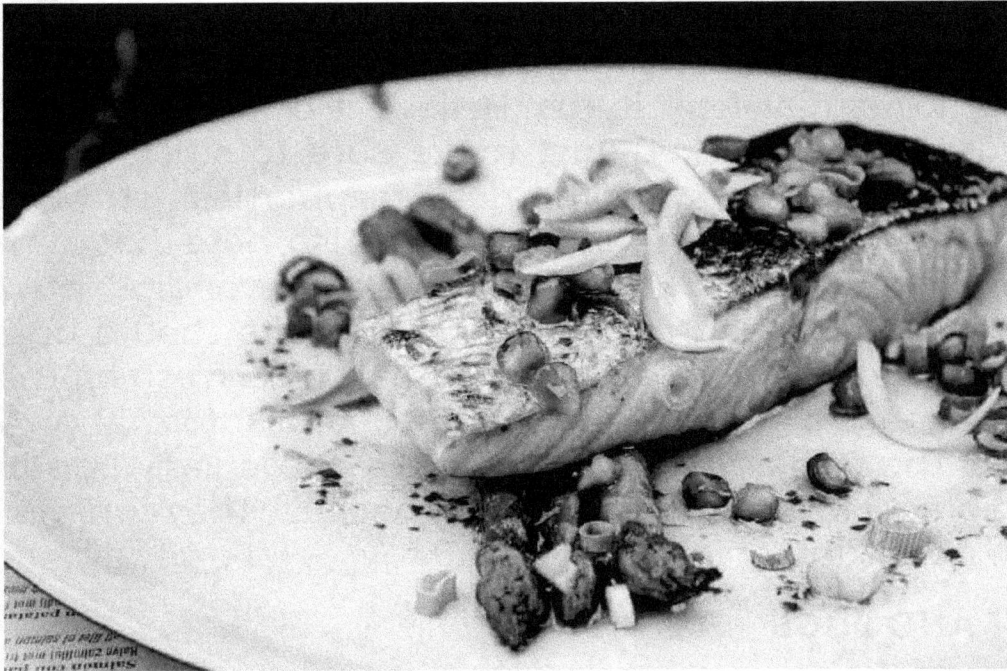

SEAFOOD

Seafood means fish like sardines, mackerel, and wild salmon. It's also a good idea to add some shrimp, tuna, mussels, and crab into your diet. This is going to be a tad expensive, but worth it in the long run. What's the common denominator in all these food items? The secret is omega-3 fatty acids, which are credited for lots of health benefits. You want to add food rich in omega-3 fatty acids in your diet.

LOW-CARB VEGETABLES

Not all vegetables are good for you when it comes to the Ketogenic Diet. The vegetable choices should be limited to those with low carbohydrate counts. Pack up your cart with items like spinach, eggplant, arugula, broccoli, and cauliflower. You can also put in bell peppers, cabbage, celery, kale, Brussels sprouts, mushrooms, zucchini, and fennel.

FRUITS LOW IN SUGAR

During an episode of sugar-craving, it's usually a good idea to pick low-sugar fruit items. Believe it or not, there are lots of those in the market! Just make sure to stock up on any of these: avocado, blackberries, raspberries, strawberries, blueberries, lime, lemon, and coconut. Also, note that tomatoes are fruits too, so feel free to make side dishes or dips with loads of tomatoes! Keep in mind that these fruits should be eaten fresh and not out of a can. If you do eat them fresh off the can, however, take a good look at the nutritional information at the back of the packaging. Avocadoes are particularly popular for those practicing the Ketogenic Diet because they contain LOTS of the good kind of fat.

MEAT AND EGGS

While some diets will tell you to skip the meat, the Ketogenic Diet encourages its consumption. Meat is packed with protein that will feed your muscles and give you a consistent energy source. It's a slow but sure burn when you eat protein as opposed to carbohydrates, which are burned faster and therefore stored faster if you don't use them immediately.

But what kind of meat should you be eating? There's chicken, beef, pork, venison, turkey, and lamb. Keep in mind that quality plays a huge role here – you should be eating grass-fed organic beef or organic poultry if you want to make the most out of this food variety. The organic option lets you limit the possibility of ingesting toxins in your body due to the production process of these products. Plus, the preservation process also means added salt or sugar in the meat, which can throw off the whole diet.

NUTS AND SEEDS

Nuts and seeds you should add in your cart include chia seeds, brazil nuts, macadamia nuts, flaxseed, walnuts, hemp seeds, pecans, sesame seeds, almonds, hazelnut, and pumpkin seeds. They also contain lots of protein and very little sugar, so they're great if you have the munchies. They're the ideal snack because they're quick, easy, and will keep you full. They're high in calories, though, which is why lots of people steer clear of them. As I mentioned earlier, the Ketogenic Diet has nothing to do with calories and everything to do with the nutrient you're eating. Don't pay too much attention to the calorie count, and just remember that they're a good source of fats and protein.

DAIRY PRODUCTS

Some people in their 50s already have a hard time processing dairy products, but for those who don't – you can happily add many of these to your diet. Make sure to consume sufficient amounts of cheese, plain Greek yogurt, cream butter, and cottage cheese. These dairy products are packed with calcium, protein, and a healthy kind of fat.

OILS

Nope, we're not talking about essentials oils but rather MCT oil, coconut oil, avocado oil, nut oils, and even extra-virgin olive oil. You can start using those for your frying needs to create healthier food options. The beauty of these oils is that they add flavor to the food, making sure you don't get bored quickly with the recipes. Try picking up different types of Keto-friendly oils to add some variety to your cooking.

COFFEE AND TEA

The good news is that you don't have to skip coffee if you're going on a Ketogenic Diet. The bad news is that you can't go to Starbucks anymore and order their blended coffee choices. Instead, beverages would be limited to unsweetened tea or unsweetened coffee to keep sugar consumption low. Opt for organic coffee and tea products to make the most out of these powerful antioxidants.

DARK CHOCOLATE

Yes – chocolate is still on the menu, but it is limited to just dark chocolate. Technically, this means eating chocolate that is 70 percent cacao, which would make the taste a bit bitter.

SUGAR SUBSTITUTES

Later in the recipes part of this book, you might be surprised at some of the ingredients required in the list. This is because while sweeteners are an important part of food preparation, you can't just use any kind of sugar in your recipe. Remember: the typical sugar is pure carbohydrate. Even if you're not eating carbohydrates, if you're dumping lots of sugar in your food – you're not following the Ketogenic Diet principles.

So what do you do? You find sugar substitutes. The good news is that there are LOTS of those in the market. You can get rid of the old sugar and use any of these as a good substitute.

Stevia. This is perhaps the most familiar one in this list. It's a natural sweetener derived from plants and contains very few calories. Unlike your typical sugar, stevia may help lower the sugar levels instead of causing it to spike. Note, though, that it's sweeter than actual sugar, so when cooking with stevia, you'll need to lower the amount used. Typically, the ratio is 200 grams of sugar per 1 teaspoon of powdered stevia.

Sucralose. It contains zero calories and zero carbohydrates. It's an artificial sweetener and does not metabolize – hence the complete lack of carbohydrates. Splenda is a sweetener derived from sucralose. Note, though, that you don't want to use this as a baking substitute for sugar. Its best use is for coffee, yogurt, and oatmeal sweetening. Note that like stevia, it's also very sweet, it's 600 times sweeter than the typical sugar. Use sparingly.

Erythritol. It's a naturally occurring compound that interacts with the tongue's sweet taste receptors. Hence, it mimics the taste of sugar without actually being sugar. It does contain calories, but only about 5% of the calories you'll find in the typical sugar. Note, though, that it doesn't dissolve very well, so anything prepared with this sweetener will have a gritty feeling. This can be problematic if you're using the product for baking. As for sweetness, the typical ratio is 1 1/3 cup for 1 cup of sugar.

Xylitol. Like erythritol, xylitol is a type of sugar alcohol that's commonly used in sugar-free gum. While it still contains calories, the calories are just 3 per gram. It's a sweetener that's good for diabetic patients because it doesn't raise the body's sugar levels or insulin. The great thing about this is that you don't have to do any computations when using it for baking, cooking, or fixing a drink. The ratio of it with sugar is 1 to 1, so you can quickly make the substitution in the recipe.

WHAT ABOUT CONDIMENTS?

Condiments are still on the table, but they won't be as tasty as you're used to. Your options include mustard, olive oil mayonnaise, oil-based salad dressings, and unsweetened ketchup. Of all these condiments, ketchup is the one with the most sugar, so make a point of looking for one with reduced sugar content. Or maybe avoid ketchup altogether and stick to mustard?

WHAT ABOUT SNACKS?

The good news is that there are packed snacks for those who don't have the time to make it themselves. Sugarless nut butters, dried seaweeds, nuts, and sugar-free jerky are all available in stores. The nuts and seeds discussed in a previous paragraph all make excellent snack options.

WHAT ABOUT LABELS?

Let's not fool ourselves into thinking that we can cook food every single day. The fact is that there will be days when there will be purchases for the sake of convenience. There are also instances when you'll have problems finding the right ingredients for a given recipe. Hence, you'll need to find substitutes for certain ingredients without losing the "Keto-friendly" vibe of the product.

So what should be done? Well, you need to learn how to read labels. Food doesn't have to be specially made to be keto-friendly. You just have to make sure that it doesn't contain any of the unfriendly nutrients or that the carbohydrate content is low enough.

Here's a step by step procedure on how to make a decision based on the labels:

1. First, take a good look at the ingredient list. You can usually find this at the bottom portion of the label and properly designated as "Ingredients."

2. The first step is to look at the sugar ingredient. If it's listed as one of the first five ingredients, that already means there's too much sugar in the product to be keto-friendly. Note, though, that sugar comes with many names. The words: glucose, fructose, maltose, lactose, dextrose, corn syrup, and more, are all indicative of sugar content. You'd want to make sure they're not listed within the first five ingredients of your

buying food product. That's one of the best things about the food industry – they're required to list ingredients in the order of quantity so that the first ones listed have more volume in the product.

3. If the food passes the "sugar" test, you should next look at the carbohydrate content.

4. You'll notice that carbohydrates are often broken down into groups. Hence, labels may indicate that total carbohydrates are 5grams. Then right below that, you can see Dietary Fiber at 1gram and sugar at 1gram. The important thing to note here is that the dietary fiber and the sugar are part of the total carbohydrates.

5. Why is this important? Well, most people count the total carbohydrates when computing their carbohydrate consumption for the day. Hence, if your goal is to eat less than 50grams of carbohydrates during the day, then you'll be computing using the 5gram amount.

6. Some people, however, make use of the "net carbohydrates" when computing their consumption. Net carbohydrates are what you get when you subtract the other carbohydrate sources from the total carbohydrates. Hence, 5 grams less 1 gram for the fiber and another gram for sugar means that you'll have 3 grams of net carbohydrates.

7. Again – why is this important? The main distinction occurs for people who have diabetes. It's all about the insulin levels. However, it's all about the 50 grams of carbohydrates limitation in your diet. However, if you want to stay on the safe side, then counting the total carbohydrates is usually the best option.

8. Look at the serving size. Most people think that the nutrition in the packet refers to all the food items in the pack – but that's not the case at all. The nutritional information is per serving, so you'd want to make sure that the carbohydrate content you picture in your head is equal to the food you usually eat in one sitting. For example, a packet of nuts contains five serving in total, each serving around 5 grams of carbohydrates. If you eat two servings in one sitting, you'll have to remember that you're consuming 10 grams instead of just 5.

Chapter 10
Two-week Keto Meal Plan for Both Women and Men Over 50

DAYS	BREAKFAST	LUNCH/DINNER	DESSERT
1	Baked Avocado Eggs	Basil Zucchini Soup	Avocado Yogurt Dip
2	Mushroom Omelet	Pesto Flavored Steak	Delicious Chocolate Frosty
3	Spicy Cream Cheese Pancakes	Beef and Broccoli	Low Carb Keto Cupcake Recipe
4	Coconut Porridge	Shredded Cilantro Lime Pork	Raspberry Mousse
5	Baked Avocado Eggs	Lamb Shanks	Quick and Simple Brownie
6	Mushroom Omelet	Nutritious Tuna Patties	Rainbow Mason Jar Salad
7	Spicy Cream Cheese Pancakes	Radish Hash Browns	Cucumber Salad with Tomatoes and Feta
8	Coconut Porridge	Yummy Chicken Skewers	Keto Macadamia Hummus

DAYS	BREAKFAST	LUNCH/DINNER	DESSERT
9	Baked Avocado Eggs	Basil Zucchini Soup	Delicious Chocolate Frosty
10	Mushroom Omelet	Pesto Flavored Steak	Low Carb Keto Cupcake Recipe
11	Spicy Cream Cheese Pancakes	Beef and Broccoli	Raspberry Mousse
12	Coconut Porridge	Shredded Cilantro Lime Pork	Quick and Simple Brownie
13	Baked Avocado Eggs	Lamb Shanks	Delicious Chocolate Frosty
14	Mushroom Omelet	Nutritious Tuna Patties	Cucumber Salad with Tomatoes and Feta

BREAKFAST

Baked Avocado Eggs

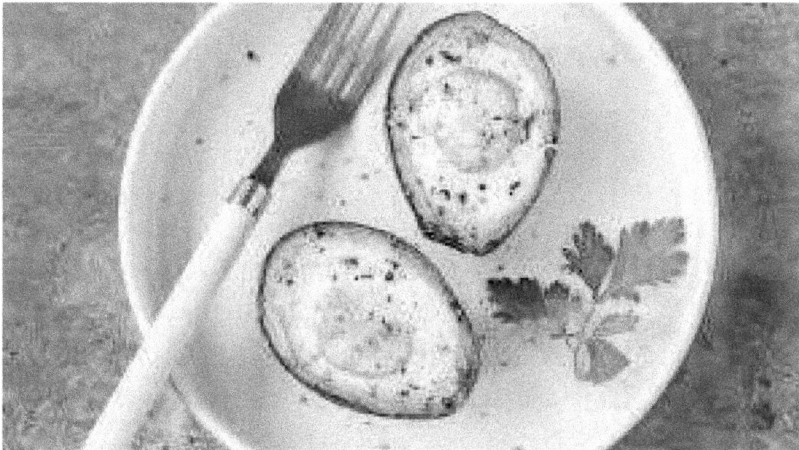

This recipe is very simple. Usually, when I buy fresh avocado, I always try to cook it simply.

Preparation Time: 10 minutes

Cooking Time: 20 minutes

Servings: 2

Ingredients:

- 2 avocados
- 4 eggs
- ½ cup bacon bits, around 55 grams
- 2 tbsp. fresh chives, chopped
- 1 sprig of chopped fresh basil, chopped
- 1 cherry tomato, quartered
- Salt and pepper to taste
- Shredded cheddar cheese

Directions:

1. Start by preheating the oven to 400 degrees Fahrenheit
2. Slice the avocado and remove the pits. Put them on a baking sheet and crack some eggs onto the center hole of the avocado. If it's too small, just scoop out more of the flesh to make room. Salt and pepper to taste.
3. Top with bacon bits and bake for 15 minutes.
4. Remove and sprinkle with herbs. Enjoy!

Nutrition:

Contains around 271 calories, 21g of fat, 7g fat, 5g fiber, 13g protein, and 7g carbohydrates

Mushroom Omelet

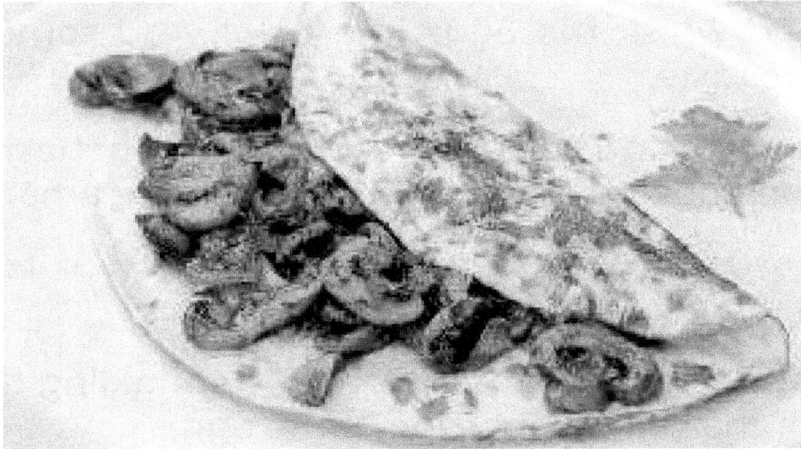

A great option for a wholesome, fun, and easy breakfast.

Preparation Time: 10 minutes

Cooking Time: 40 minutes

Servings: 2

Ingredients:

- 3 eggs, medium
- 1 oz. shredded cheese
- 1 oz. butter used for frying
- ¼ yellow onion, chopped
- 4 large sliced mushrooms
- Your favorite vegetables, optional
- Salt and pepper to taste

Directions:

1. Crack and whisk the eggs in a bowl. Add some salt and pepper to taste.

2. Melt the butter in a pan using low heat. Put in the mushroom and onion, cooking the two until you get that amazing smell.

3. Pour the egg mix into the pan and allow it to cook on medium heat.

4. Allow the bottom part to cook before sprinkling the cheese on top of the still-raw portion of the egg.

5. Carefully pry the edges of the omelet and fold it in half. Allow it to cook for a few seconds before removing the pan from the heat and sliding it directly onto your plate.

Nutrition:

5 grams of carbohydrates, 1 gram of fiber, 44 grams of fat, 26 grams of protein, and 520 kcalories.

Spicy Cream Cheese Pancakes

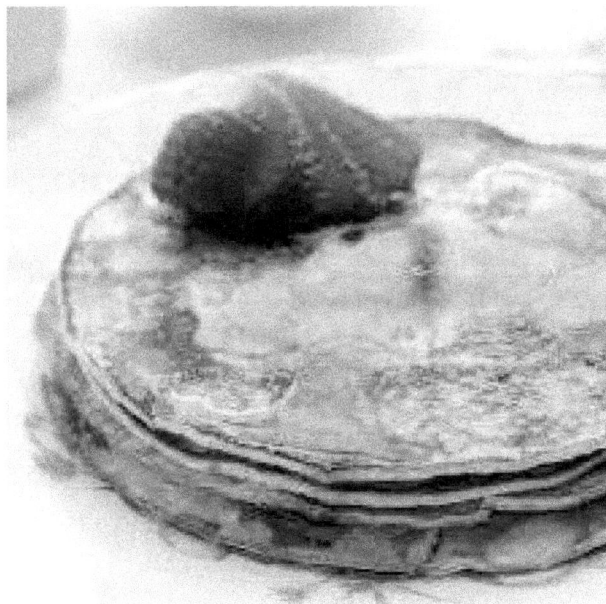

It's a delicious breakfast you need to try soon!

Preparation Time: 10 minutes

Cooking Time: 60 minutes

Servings: 2

Ingredients:

- 3 eggs
- 9 Tbsp cottage cheese
- Salt, to taste
- ½ Tbsp psyllium husk powder
- Butter, for frying
- 4 oz cream cheese
- 1 Tbsp green pesto
- 1 Tbsp olive oil

- ¼ red onion, finely sliced
- Black pepper, to taste

Directions:

1. Combine cream cheese, olive oil, and pesto. Put this mixture aside.

2. Blend eggs, psyllium husk powder, cottage cheese, and salt until the mixture is smooth. Leave it for 5 minutes.

3. Heat the butter in the pan and put several dollops of cottage cheese batter into the pan. Fry for a few minutes each side.

4. Top your pancakes with a large amount of cream cheese mixture and several red onion slices.

5. Add black pepper and olive oil.

Nutrition:

Carbohydrates 7 g, Fat 38 g, Protein 18 g, Calories 449

Coconut Porridge

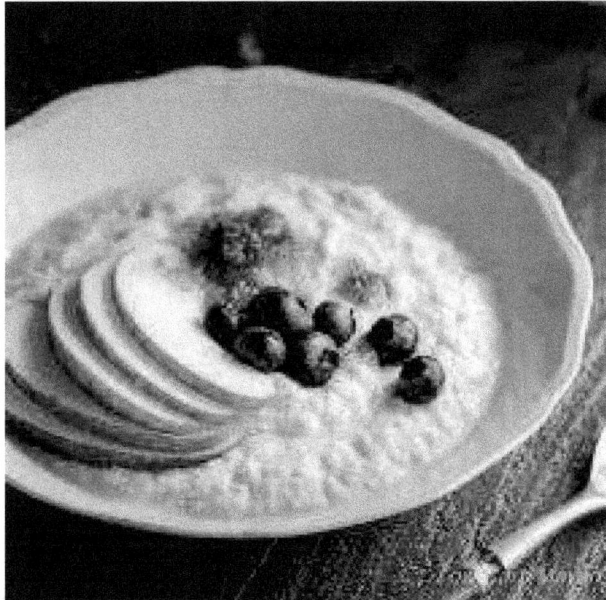

It's not only extremely tasty! It is also easy to make.

Preparation Time: 10 minutes

Cooking Time: 50 minutes

Servings: 2

Ingredients:

- Shredded coconut, unsweetened – 1 cup
- Coconut milk, unsweetened and full-fat – 2 cups
- Water – 2 2/3 cups
- Coconut flour – 1/4 cup
- Psyllium husks – 1/4 cup
- Vanilla extract, unsweetened – 1 teaspoon
- Cinnamon – 1/2 teaspoon

- Nutmeg – 1/4 teaspoon

- Stevia, liquid – 30 drops

- Monk fruit sweetener, liquid – 20 drops

Directions:

1. Switch on the instant pot, press the 'sauté/simmer' button, wait until hot, add the coconut and cook for 3 minutes or more until toast.

2. Pour in water and milk, stir well and press the 'keep warm' button.

3. Shut the instant pot with its lid in the sealed position, then press the 'manual' button, press '+/-' to set the cooking time to 10 minutes and cook at high-pressure setting; when the pressure builds in the pot, the cooking timer will start.

4. When the instant pot buzzes, press the 'keep warm' button, release pressure naturally for 10 minutes, then do a quick pressure release and open the lid.

5. Add remaining ingredients, stir well and serve.

Nutrition:

Calories 303, Fat 25 g, Protein 3 g, Net Carbs 10 g, Fiber 11 g

LUNCH

Basil Zucchini Soup

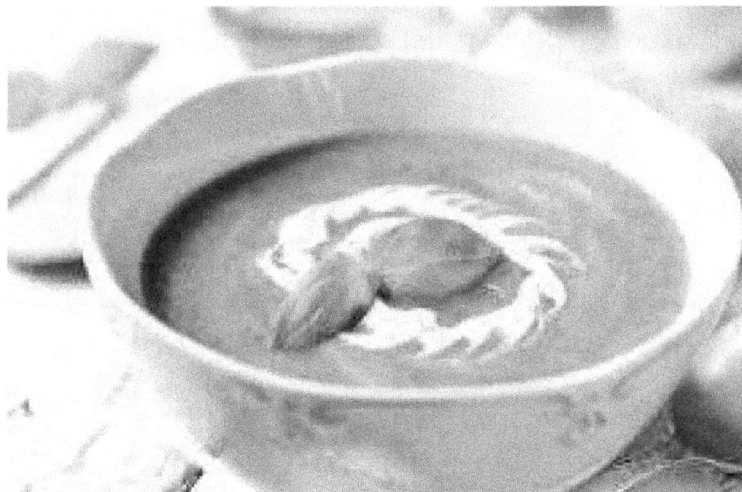

It's a delicious soup you need to try soon!

Preparation Time: 10 minutes

Cooking Time: 25 minutes

Servings: 4

Ingredients:

- 2 medium zucchinis, chopped
- ¼ cup fresh basil leaves
- 3 cups vegetable broth
- 3 tbsp olive oil
- 1 tbsp garlic, chopped
- 1 medium onion, chopped
- ¼ tsp pepper
- ½ tsp salt

Directions:

1. Heat olive oil in a saucepan over medium heat.

2. Add garlic and onion and sauté for 3-5 minutes or until onion is softened.

3. Add zucchini and cook for 5 minutes.

4. Add stock and bring to boil. Turn heat to low and simmer for 15 minutes.

5. Remove from heat. Add basil and stir well.

6. Puree the soup using an immersion blender until smooth.

7. Season soup with pepper and salt.

8. Serve and enjoy.

Nutrition:

Calories 149, Fat 11.8 g, Carbohydrates 7.3 g, Sugar 3.4 g, Protein 5.3 g

Pesto Flavored Steak

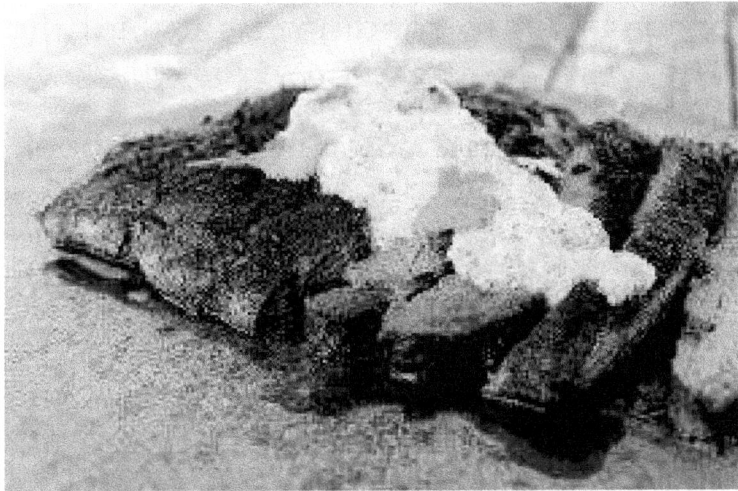

If you are looking for a new dish to try with the family, try this pesto flavored steak.

Preparation Time: 15 minutes

Cooking Time: 17 minutes

Servings: 4

Ingredients:

- ¼ C. fresh oregano, chopped
- 1½ tbsp. garlic, minced
- 1 tbsp. fresh lemon peel, grated
- ½ tsp. red pepper flakes, crushed
- Salt and freshly ground black pepper, to taste
- 1 lb. (1-inch thick) grass-fed boneless beef top sirloin steak
- 1 C. pesto
- ¼ C. feta cheese, crumbled

Directions:

1. Preheat the gas grill to medium heat. Lightly, grease the grill grate.

2. In a bowl, add the oregano, garlic, lemon peel, red pepper flakes, salt, and black pepper and mix well.

3. Rub the garlic mixture onto the steak evenly.

4. Place the steak on the grill and cook, covered for about 12-17 minutes, flipping occasionally.

5. Remove from the grill and place the steak onto a cutting board for about 5 minutes.

6. With a sharp knife, cut the steak into desired sized slices.

7. Divide the steak slices and pesto onto serving plates and serve with the topping of the feta cheese.

Nutrition:

Calories 226, Carbohydrates 6.8g, Protein 40.5g, Fat 7.6g, Sugar 0.7g, Sodium 579mg, Fiber 2.2g

Beef and Broccoli

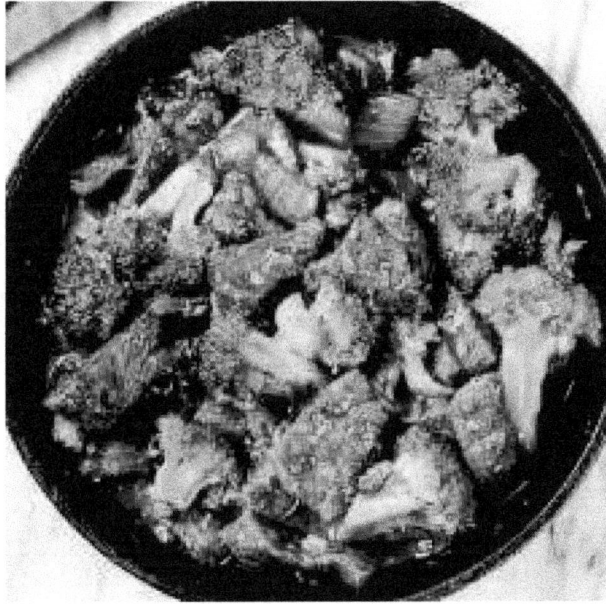

This dish is sure to delight the whole family. It will warm you from the inside out with every bite.

Preparation Time: 5 minutes

Cooking Time: 25 minutes

Servings: 4

Ingredients:

- Chuck roast, sliced – 1 ½ pound

- Broccoli florets – 12 ounces

- Garlic cloves, peeled – 4

- Avocado oil – 2 tablespoons

- Soy sauce – ½ cup

- Erythritol sweetener – ¼ cup

- Xanthan gum – 1 tablespoon

Directions:

1. Switch on the instant pot, grease pot with oil, press the 'sauté/simmer' button, wait until the oil is hot and add the beef slices and garlic and cook for 5 to 10 minutes or until browned.

2. Meanwhile, whisk together sweetener, soy sauce, and broth until combined.

3. Pour sauce over browned beef, toss it until well coated, press the 'keep warm' button, and shut the instant pot with its lid in the sealed position.

4. Press the 'manual' button, press '+/-' to set the cooking time to 10 minutes, and cook at a high-pressure setting; when the pressure builds in the pot, the cooking timer will start.

5. Meanwhile, place broccoli florets in a large heatproof bowl, cover with plastic wrap and microwave for 4 minutes, or until tender.

6. When the instant pot buzzes, press the 'keep warm' button, do a quick pressure release and open the lid.

7. Take out ¼ cup of cooking liquid, stir in xanthan gum until combined, then add into the instant pot and stir until mixed.

8. Press the 'sauté/simmer' button and simmer beef and sauce for 5 minutes or until it reaches the desired consistency.

9. Then add broccoli florets, stir until mixed and press the cancel button.

10. Serve broccoli and beef with cauliflower rice.

Nutrition:

Calories 351.4, Fat 12.4 g, Protein 29 g, Net Carbs 11 g, Fiber 8 g

Shredded Cilantro Lime Pork

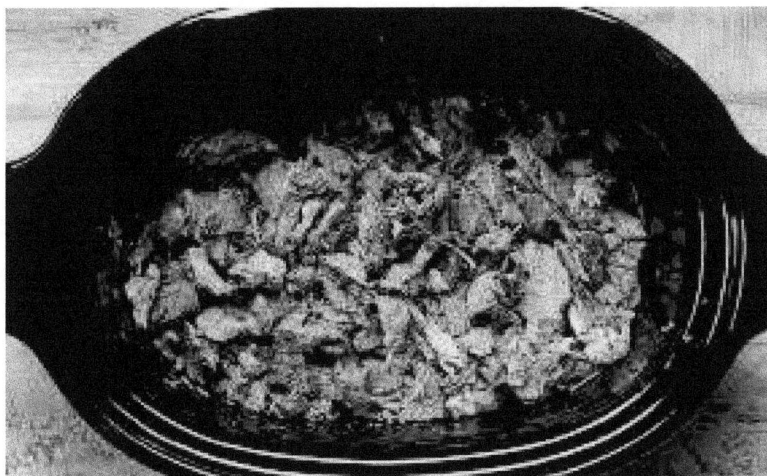

Preparation Time: 10 minutes

Cooking Time: 6 hours

Servings: 6

Ingredients:

- 2 lbs. pork sirloin roast
- ¼ tsp garlic powder
- ¼ cup fresh cilantro, chopped
- ½ tbsp cumin
- 1 ½ tbsp chili powder
- ¼ cup fresh lime juice
- 1 ½ tsp kosher salt

Directions:

1. Place pork into the slow cooker.

2. Add remaining ingredients on top of the pork.

3. Cover slow cooker with lid and cook on low for 6 hours.

4. Remove pork from slow cooker and shred using a fork.

5. Return shredded pork to the slow cooker and stir well.

6. Serve and enjoy.

Nutrition:

Calories 321, Fat 14.7g, Carbohydrates 1.3 g, Sugar 0.2 g, Protein 43.4 g, Cholesterol 130 mg

DINNER

Lamb Shanks

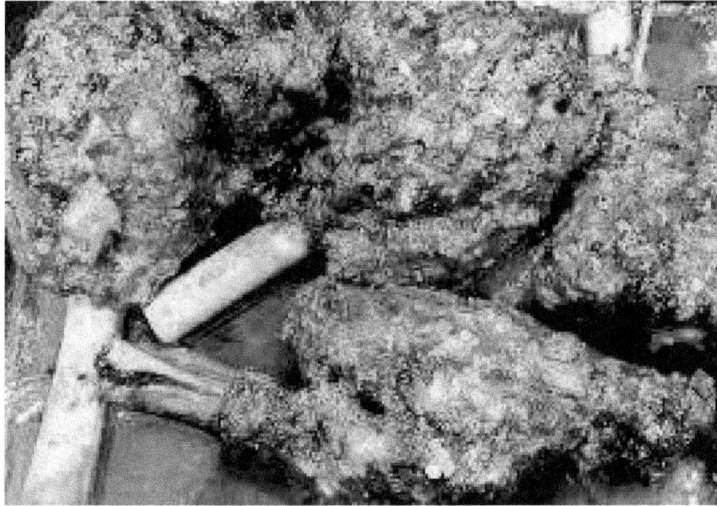

It's always a pleasure to discover such a wonderful lunch!

Preparation Time: 10 minutes

Cooking Time: 30 minutes

Servings: 2

Ingredients:

- Avocado oil – 1/4 cup
- Lamb shanks – 2.5 pounds
- Minced garlic – 1 tablespoon
- Medium white onion, peeled and diced – 1
- Sticks of celery, diced – 2
- Rosemary – 2 tablespoons
- Salt – 1 teaspoon

- Ground black pepper – 1/2 teaspoon

- Lamb or chicken broth – 1 cup

- Diced tomatoes – 14 ounces

Directions:

1. Switch on the instant pot, add half of the oil, press the 'sauté/ simmer' button, wait until the oil is hot and lamb shanks in a single layer, and cook for 3 to 5 minutes per side or until browned.

2. Transfer lamb shanks to a plate, set aside, then add onion, celery, garlic, and rosemary into the instant pot and cook for 3 minutes.

3. Season with salt and black pepper, pour in the broth, mix well, add tomatoes, and return lamb shanks into the pot and toss until combined.

4. Press the 'keep warm' button, shut the instant pot with its lid in the sealed position, then press the 'manual' button, press '+/-' to set the cooking time to 50 minutes and cook at high-pressure setting; when the pressure builds in the pot, the cooking timer will start.

5. When the instant pot buzzes, press the 'keep warm' button, release pressure naturally for 10 minutes, then do a quick pressure release and open the lid.

6. Transfer lamb shanks to a dish, press the 'sauté/simmer' button, and simmer it for 5 minutes or more until the sauce is reduced by half.

7. Ladle sauce over the lamb shanks and serve.

Nutrition:

Calories 410, Fat 35 g, Protein 51 g, Net Carbs 12 g, Fiber 3 g

Nutritious Tuna Patties

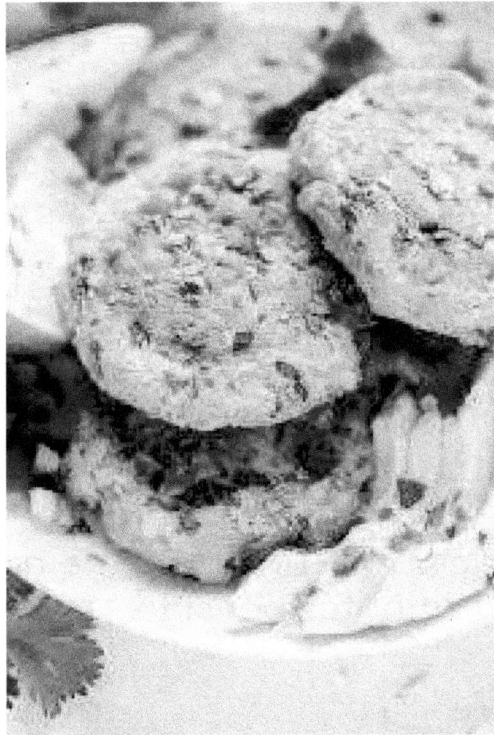

A great option for a wholesome, fun, and easy dinner.

Preparation Time: 10 minutes

Cooking Time: 15 minutes

Servings: 8

Ingredients:

- 2 cans tuna, drained and flaked
- 4 tbsp olive oil
- ¼ cup fresh parsley, chopped
- 2 eggs, lightly beaten
- 3 garlic cloves, minced

- 2 tbsp Dijon mustard
- 2 tbsp mayonnaise
- ¼ tsp pepper
- ½ tsp salt

Directions:

1. Preheat the oven to 170 F.

2. In a bowl, mix tuna, parsley, eggs, garlic, Dijon mustard, mayonnaise, pepper, and salt.

3. Heat oil in a pan over medium heat.

4. Make small patties from tuna mixture and fry until golden brown, about 2-3 minutes per side.

5. Serve and enjoy.

Nutrition:

Calories 178, Fat 13.1 g, Carbohydrates 1.7 g, Sugar 0.4 g,

Protein 13.5 g, Cholesterol 56 mg

Radish Hash Browns

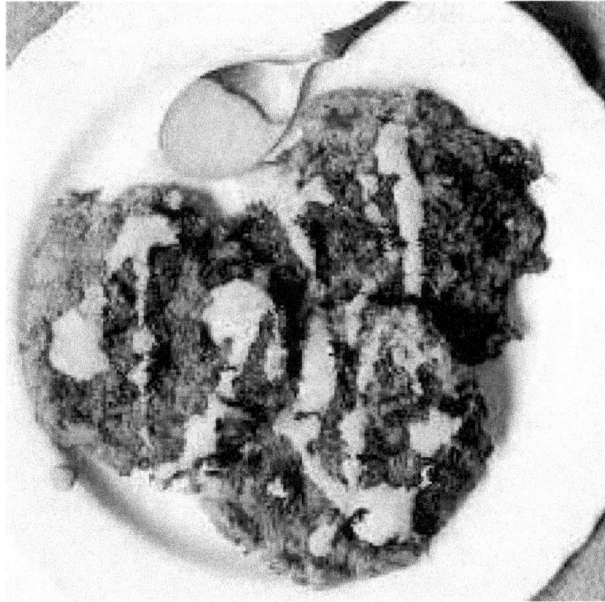

If you are looking for a new dish to try with the family, try these radish hash browns.

Preparation Time: 10 minutes

Cooking Time: 10 minutes

Servings: 4

Ingredients:

- Onion powder – ½ tsp.

- Radishes – 1 pound, shredded

- Garlic powder – ½ tsp.

- Salt and ground black pepper to taste

- Eggs – 4

- Parmesan cheese – 1/3 cup, grated

Directions:

1. In a bowl, mix radishes, with salt, pepper, onion, garlic powder, eggs, Parmesan cheese, and mix well.

2. Spread on a lined baking sheet.

3. Place in an oven at 375F and bake for 10 minutes.

4. Serve.

Nutrition:

Calories 104, Fat 6g, Carb 4.5g, Protein 8.6g, Sodium 276 mg

Yummy Chicken Skewers

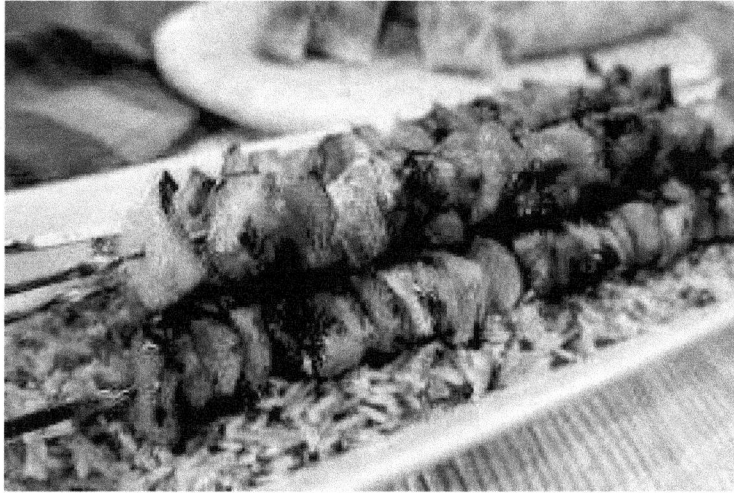

Preparation Time: 10 minutes

Cooking Time: 10 minutes

Servings: 8

Ingredients:

- 2 lbs. chicken breast tenderloins
- 1 tsp lemon pepper seasoning
- 1 tsp garlic, minced
- 1 tbsp olive oil
- 1 cup of salsa

Directions:

1. Add chicken in a zip-lock bag along with 1/4 cup salsa, lemon pepper seasoning, garlic, and oil.

2. Seal bag and shake well and place it in the refrigerator overnight.

3. Thread marinated chicken onto the soaked wooden skewers.

4. Place skewers on hot grill and cooks for 8-10 minutes.

5. Brush with remaining salsa during the last 3 minutes of grilling.

6. Serve and enjoy.

Nutrition:

Calories 125, Fat 2.5 g, Carbohydrates 2.1 g, Sugar 1 g, Protein 24 g, Cholesterol 71 mg

APPETIZER

Avocado Yogurt Dip

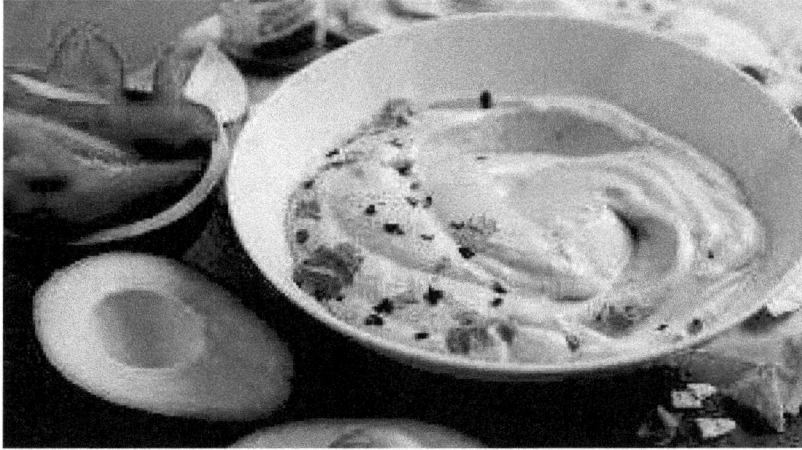

Everyone in your family will want to add this dish to your regular weekly meals.

Preparation Time: 5 minutes

Cooking Time: 5 minutes

Servings: 4

Ingredients:

- 2 avocados
- 1 lime juice
- 3 garlic cloves, minced
- ½ cup Greek yogurt
- Pepper
- Salt

Directions:

1. Scoop out avocado flesh using the spoon and place it in a bowl.

2. Mash avocado flesh using the fork.

3. Add remaining ingredients and stir to combine.

4. Serve and enjoy.

Nutrition:

Calories 139, Fat 11 g, Carbohydrates 9 g, Protein 4 g, Sugar 2g, Cholesterol 15 mg

Rainbow Mason Jar Salad

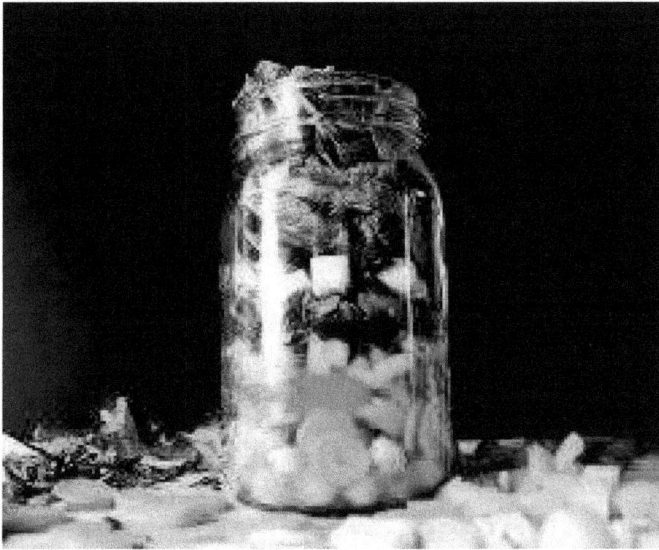

Rainbow Mason Jar Salad has always been a favorite among many people, and it is quite easy to make.

Preparation Time: 10 minutes

Cooking Time: 30 minutes

Servings: 4

Ingredients:

- Arugula, fresh – 1/2 cup
- Medium radishes, sliced – 2
- Medium yellow squash, spiralized – 1/4
- Butternut squash, peeled, cubed – 1/4 cup
- Fresh blueberries – 1/4 cup
- Avocado oil – 1 tablespoon

The Dressing:

- Medium avocado, peeled, cubed – 1/4
- Avocado oil – 2 tablespoons
- Apple cider vinegar – 1 tablespoon
- Filtered water – 1 tablespoon
- Cilantro leaves – 1 tablespoon
- Salt – 1/4 teaspoon

Directions:

1. Set oven to 350 degrees F and let preheat.
2. Then place cubes of butternut squash in a bowl, drizzle with oil, toss until well coated and then spread evenly on a baking sheet.
3. Place the baking sheet into the oven and bake for 30 minutes or until tender.
4. Meanwhile, prepare the salad dressing. For this, place all the ingredients for the dressing in a blender and pulse for 1 to 2 minutes or until smooth, set aside until required.
5. When the butternut squash is baked, take out the baking sheet from the oven and let squash cool for 15 minutes.
6. Then take a 32-ounce mason jar, pour in the prepared dressing, layer with radish, and top with roasted butternut squash, squash noodles, berries, and arugula.
7. Seal the jar and store in the refrigerator for up to 5 days.

Nutrition:

Calories 516, Fat 49 g, Protein 2 g, Net Carbs 6 g, Fiber 6 g

Cucumber Salad with Tomatoes and Feta

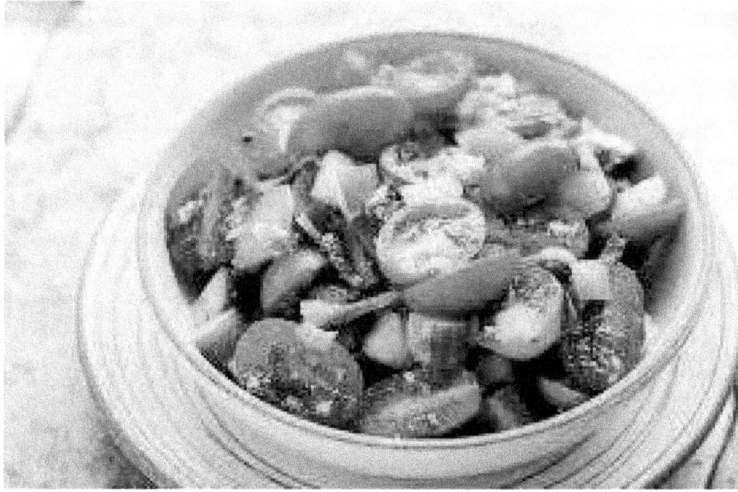

This is a great recipe for anyone who loves tomatoes.

Preparation Time: 15 minutes

Cooking Time: 0 minutes

Servings: 4

Ingredients:

- 2 cucumbers, diced
- 6 tomatoes, diced
- ¾ cup feta cheese, crumbled
- ½ white onion, chopped
- 1 clove garlic, minced
- 2 Tbsp lime juice
- 2 Tbsp parsley, chopped
- 2 Tbsp dill, chopped
- 3 Tbsp olive oil

- 3 Tbsp red wine vinegar
- Salt and black pepper, to taste

Directions:

1. Combine all the ingredients in a bowl.
2. Stir thoroughly and serve.

Nutrition:

Carbohydrates 5 g, fat 10 g, Protein 3 g, Calories 125

Keto Macadamia Hummus

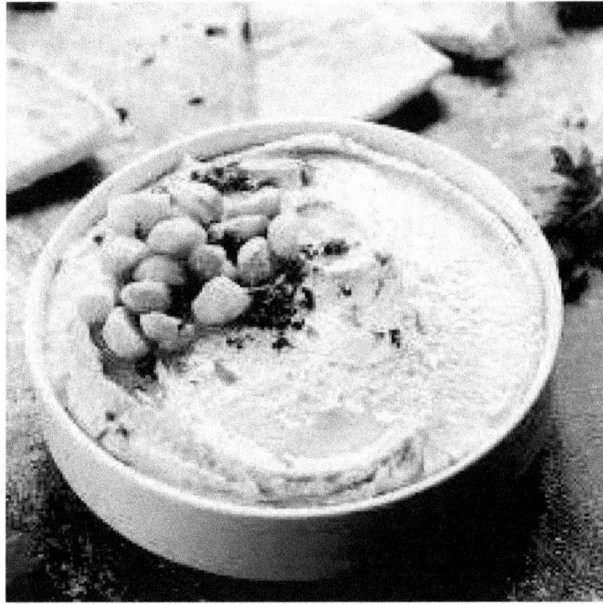

This is a great dish for any occasion. It is very hearty. You can serve this alongside a salad and some milk to complete a nice lunch.

Preparation Time: 10 minutes

Cooking Time: 5 minutes

Servings: 8

Ingredients:

- 1 cup macadamia nuts, soaked in water for overnight, drained and rinsed
- 1 ½ tbsp tahini
- 2 tbsp water
- 2 tbsp fresh lime juice
- 2 garlic cloves

- 1/8 tsp cayenne pepper
- Pepper
- Salt

Directions:

1. Add all ingredients into the food processor and process until smooth.

2. Serve and enjoy.

Nutrition:

Calories 138, Fat 14.2 g, Carbohydrates 3.2 g, Protein 1.9 g,

Sugar 1.9 g, Cholesterol 0 mg

DESERT

Delicious Chocolate Frosty

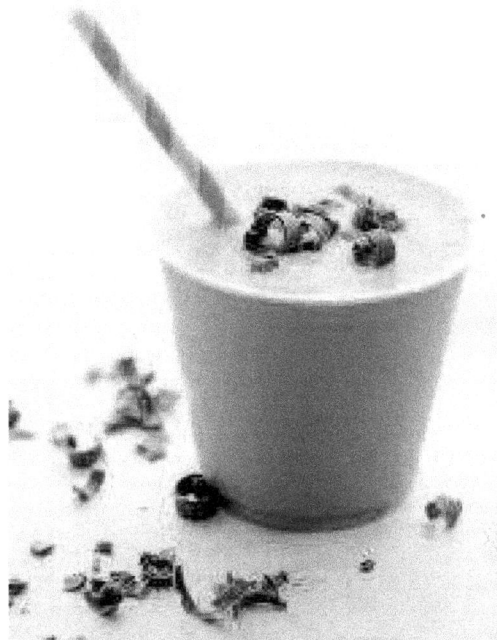

This is not only sweet, but it tastes wonderful.

Preparation Time: 10 minutes

Cooking Time: 10 minutes

Servings: 2

Ingredients:

- 1 ½ cups heavy whipping cream
- 2 ½ tbsp lakanto monk fruit
- 1 tbsp vanilla
- 2 tbsp unsweetened cocoa powder

Directions:

1. Add all ingredients into the large mixing bowl.

2. Beat using the hand mixer until peaks form.

3. Scoop mixture into the zip-lock bag and place it in the refrigerator for 45 minutes.

4. Remove a zip-lock bag from the refrigerator and cut the corner of the bag.

5. Squeeze frosty in serving bowls. Serve chilled.

Nutrition:

Calories 342, Fat 34 g, Carbohydrates 6.3 g, Sugar 1 g,

Protein 2.9 g, Cholesterol 123 mg

Low Carb Keto Cupcake Recipe

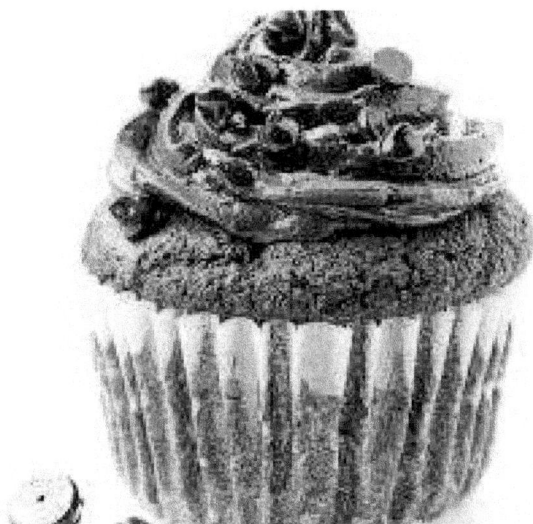

This dish is packed full of nutrients. You can now enjoy it at any time of the year.

Preparation Time: 10 minutes

Cooking Time: 40 minutes

Servings: 2

Ingredients:

- 4 eggs
- 1/3 cup coconut flour
- ½ cup unsweetened cocoa powder
- ¼ cup powdered erythritol
- 1 tsp. baking powder
- ½ tsp baking soda
- ¼ tsp. salt
- 1 tsp. vanilla extract

- 4 tbsp. extra light olive oil

- ½ cup unsweetened almond milk

Directions:

1. Start by preheating oven the 350 degrees Fahrenheit. Grab the muffin tin and grease is up or put the cupcake liners while waiting.

2. Grab a bowl and combine the cocoa powder, coconut flour, baking powder, baking soda, salt, and erythritol. Whisk all the ingredients thoroughly.

3. Add the eggs, vanilla extract, almond oil, and olive oil. Mix completely until they're well combined. Allow it to sit for 5 minutes. Check to see if the mixture has the desired thickness. If not, you can add water until it gets the thickness you want. Make sure to add one tablespoon at a time to help control the amount.

4. Put around 2 tablespoons of the batter into the muffin tin.

5. Bake for 20 minutes or until a toothpick comes out clean after inserting it in the center of the muffin.

Nutrition:

66 kcalories, 45g fat, 16g saturated fat, 1mg cholesterol, 88mg potassium, 2g fiber, and 1g protein

Raspberry Mousse

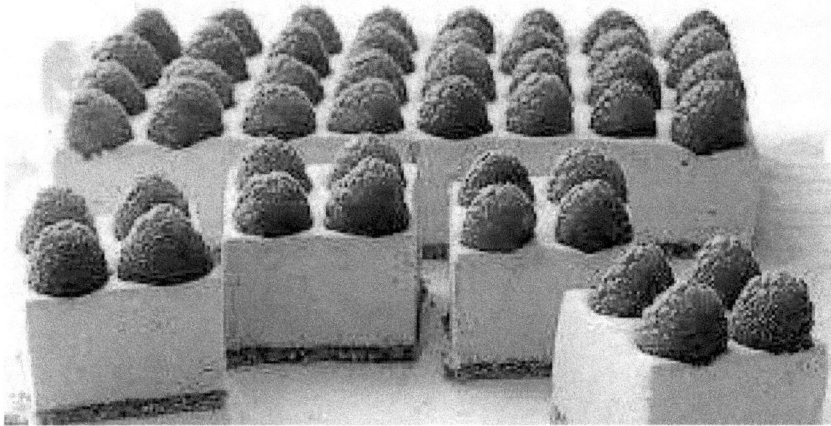

This is the perfect recipe for anyone who is looking to please their family or a crowd.

Preparation Time: 10 minutes

Cooking Time: 4 hours

Servings: 8

Ingredients:

- 3 oz fresh raspberry
- 2 cups heavy whipping cream
- 2 oz pecans, chopped
- ¼ tsp vanilla extract
- ½ lemon, the zest

Directions:

1. Pour the whipping cream into the dish and blend until it becomes soft.

2. Put the lemon zest and vanilla into the dish and mix thoroughly.

3. Put the raspberries and nuts into the cream mix and stir well.

4. Cover the dish with plastic wrap and put it in the fridge for 3 hours.

5. Top with raspberries and serve

Nutrition:

Carbohydrates 3 g, Fat 26 g, Protein 2 g, Calories 255

Quick and Simple Brownie

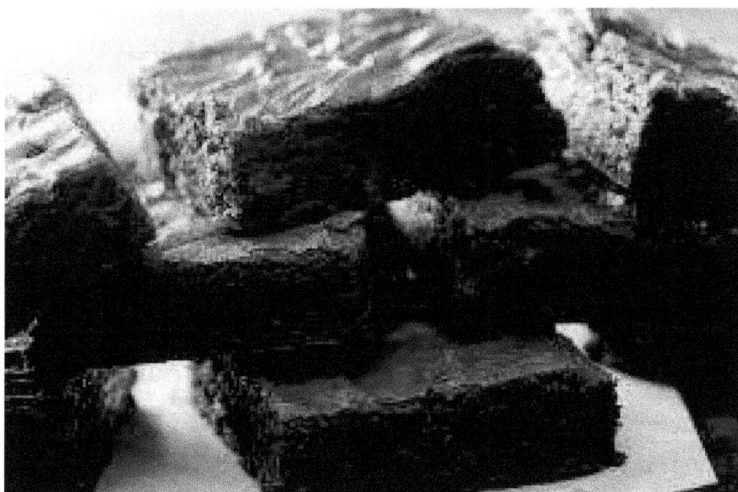

A great option for a wholesome, fun, and easy dessert.

Preparation Time: 20 minutes

Cooking Time: 5 minutes

Servings: 2

Ingredients:

- 3 Tbsp Keto chocolate chips
- 1 Tbsp unsweetened cacao powder
- 2 Tbsp salted butter
- 2¼ Tbsp powdered sugar

Directions:

1. Combine 2 Tbsp of chocolate chips and butter, melt them in a microwave for 10-15 minutes. Add the remaining chocolate chips, stir and make a sauce.

2. Add the cacao powder and powdered sugar to the sauce and whisk well until you have a dough.

3. Place the dough on a baking sheet, form the Brownie.

4. Put your Brownie into the oven (preheated to 350°F).

5. Bake for 5 minutes.

Nutrition:

Carbohydrates 9 g, Fat 30 g, Protein 13 g, Calories 100

Chapter 12

Dining Out on Keto

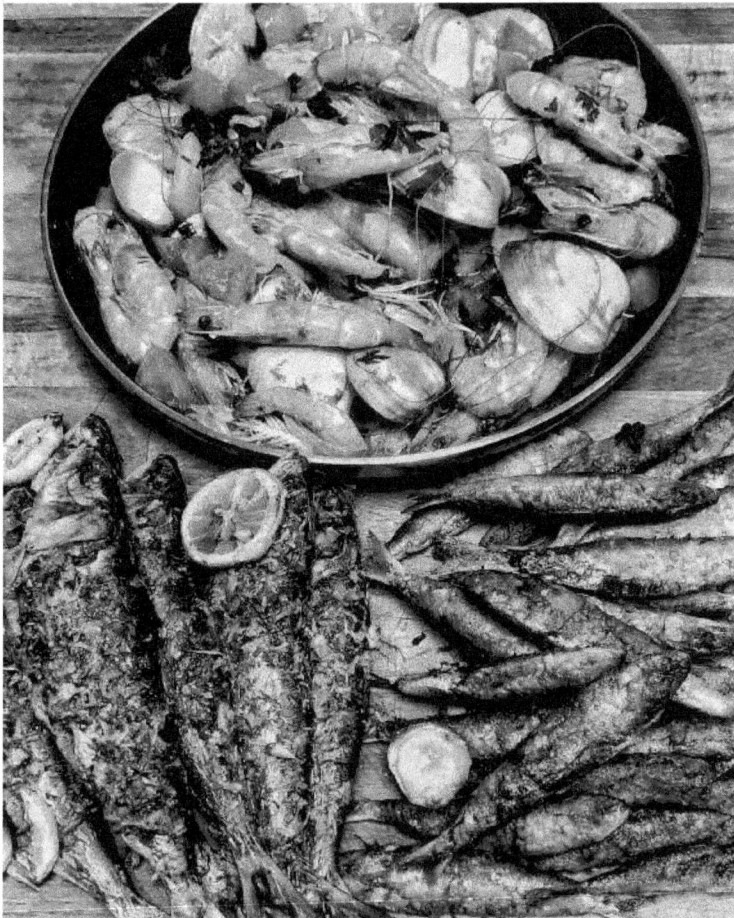

Eating out or away from home can be a challenge for those partaking in a diet plan. Keto aimed to change this perspective. It proved to people that they can still lose weight and maintain a satisfying lifestyle while doing so. Many would argue that being on Keto does not feel like a diet plan at all. Instead, it acts as a guideline for how we need to treat our bodies by providing a simple yet effective method. Keto is so enjoyable because it doesn't ask you to count calories every single day. It is a more flexible diet plan that allows individuals to still feel that they are individuals.

Depending on how much time you have in your current schedule, you might find that you would rather prepare most of your meals. There is some variety in the menus in terms of where you will be getting your food. Takeout is still a viable option if that is something that you already utilize in your normal lifestyle. A lot of people decide that Keto is a turning point, though. They often meal prep and plan well in advance to ensure that they are truly maintaining their diets. Though you can eat takeout and have meals at restaurants, you must be very careful regarding the ingredients that they are using. Modifications are almost always going to be necessary.

It is a good thing for you to be aware of these options because, sometimes, eating out is going to be your only option. Whether you are meeting with a friend for lunch or having a business meeting away from the office, there will be times when you need to eat with others. Many of us worry that being on a diet automatically means that these fun times at restaurants must come to an end and be replaced with us sitting there without a plate of food. You don't have to give up eating in its entirety to eat Keto all the time! The easiest way to eat out while on Keto is to focus on your protein. Almost any restaurant you go to will have a dish that is protein-focused.

After you've found your protein of choice, determine what sides it comes with. Anything carb-heavy can usually be replaced by veggies or something that contains dairy. Make sure that you ask about these substitutions before completely ruling out the entree. If you explain to the server what you can and cannot eat, you are likely to get some recommendations. People go out to eat while on diets all the time, and restaurants generally tend to be fairly accommodating. While you are on the Keto diet, don't be afraid to ask about modifications and substitutions. Your diet plan is important to you, so treat it that way.

If you'd rather rely on your skills to make your Keto-friendly menu, think about how to make the process even more efficient for yourself. While some people enjoy cooking every single day, others don't have the time for it. Meal prepping can help you greatly. If you can devote a single day to your grocery shopping and meal prepping, you can likely save a lot of time when it comes to how much cooking must be done. Try to plan your menus ahead of time, taking note of recipes that sound interesting and healthy. When you have these ideas in advance, you will likely be able to make faster decisions in the grocery store.

Use your meal prep time as a time to unwind. Even if cooking isn't your favorite thing to do, know that you are doing this because you are investing in your health. Prepare and store all of the food that you will need for the week, dividing it into portion-controlled containers. Ideally, you should sort all of the food by meal type. This way, you will be able to simply grab a portion and go or heat it when you need to eat something. Many Keto meal prep recipes can be eaten either hot or cold, which is helpful when you are at the office or anywhere else away from your home. You might find that the whole family will become interested in your newfound meal prep ways.

If you want to get the entire family involved in meal planning, this serves as a great way to bond and work together to develop the plan. Eating healthy can be difficult for many reasons, but it makes the process a lot easier when given options. Show your family the recipes you've come up with and those you have grown to love. Even if they are not on the Keto diet themselves, it is highly likely that they will find your meals just as delicious as you do. Keep a recipe book handy and add new recipes to it as you see them. When you are constantly keeping track of them, you will be more likely to remember them for later.

Remember that you can utilize a mix of both eating out and cooking for yourself when you are on Keto. The key is to take a look at your lifestyle and your current schedule to determine what will work best for you. Meal prepping can be a gradual process, so if you are only able to prep for a few days at a time, try it out this way. Nothing about eating should have to be an all or nothing process. The important thing is to pay attention to your body. If you notice that you don't feel as energized when you eat at restaurants, then you are likely not getting enough nutrition. The best way to truly give your body what it needs is by preparing the food yourself. When you can listen to your body, you will always know what you need next.

Chapter 13

Conversion Tables

VOLUME EQUIVALENTS (LIQUID)

US STANDARD	US STANDARD (OUNCES)	METRIC
2 tablespoons	1 fl. oz.	30 mL
¼ cup	2 fl. oz.	60 mL
½ cup	4 fl. oz.	120 mL
1 cup	8 fl. oz.	240mL
1½ cups	12 fl. oz.	355 mL
2 cups or 1 pint	16 fl. oz.	475 mL
4 cups or 1 quart	32 fl. oz.	1 L
1 gallon	128 fl. oz.	4 L

OVEN TEMPERATURES

FAHRENHEIT (°F)	CELSIUS (°C) APPROXIMATE
250 °F	120 °C
300 °F	150 °C
325 °F	165 °C
350 °F	180 °C
375 °F	190 °C
400 °F	200 °C
425 °F	220 °C
450 °F	230 °C

VOLUME EQUIVALENTS (LIQUID)

US STANDARD	METRIC (APPROXIMATE)
1/8 teaspoon	0.5 mL
¼ teaspoon	1 mL
½ teaspoon	2 mL
2/3 teaspoon	4 mL
1 teaspoon	5 mL
1 tablespoon	15 mL
¼ cup	59 mL
1/3 cup	79 mL
½ cup	118 mL
2/3 cup	156 mL
¾ cup	177 mL
1 cup	235 mL
2 cups or 1 pint	475 mL
3 cups	700 mL
4 cups or 1 quart	1 L
½ gallon	2 L
1 gallon	4 L

WEIGHT EQUIVALENTS

US STANDARD	METRIC (APPROXIMATE)
½ ounce	15 g
1 ounce	30 g
2 ounces	60 g
4 ounces	115 g
8 ounces	225 g
12 ounces	340 g
16 ounces or 1 pound	455 g

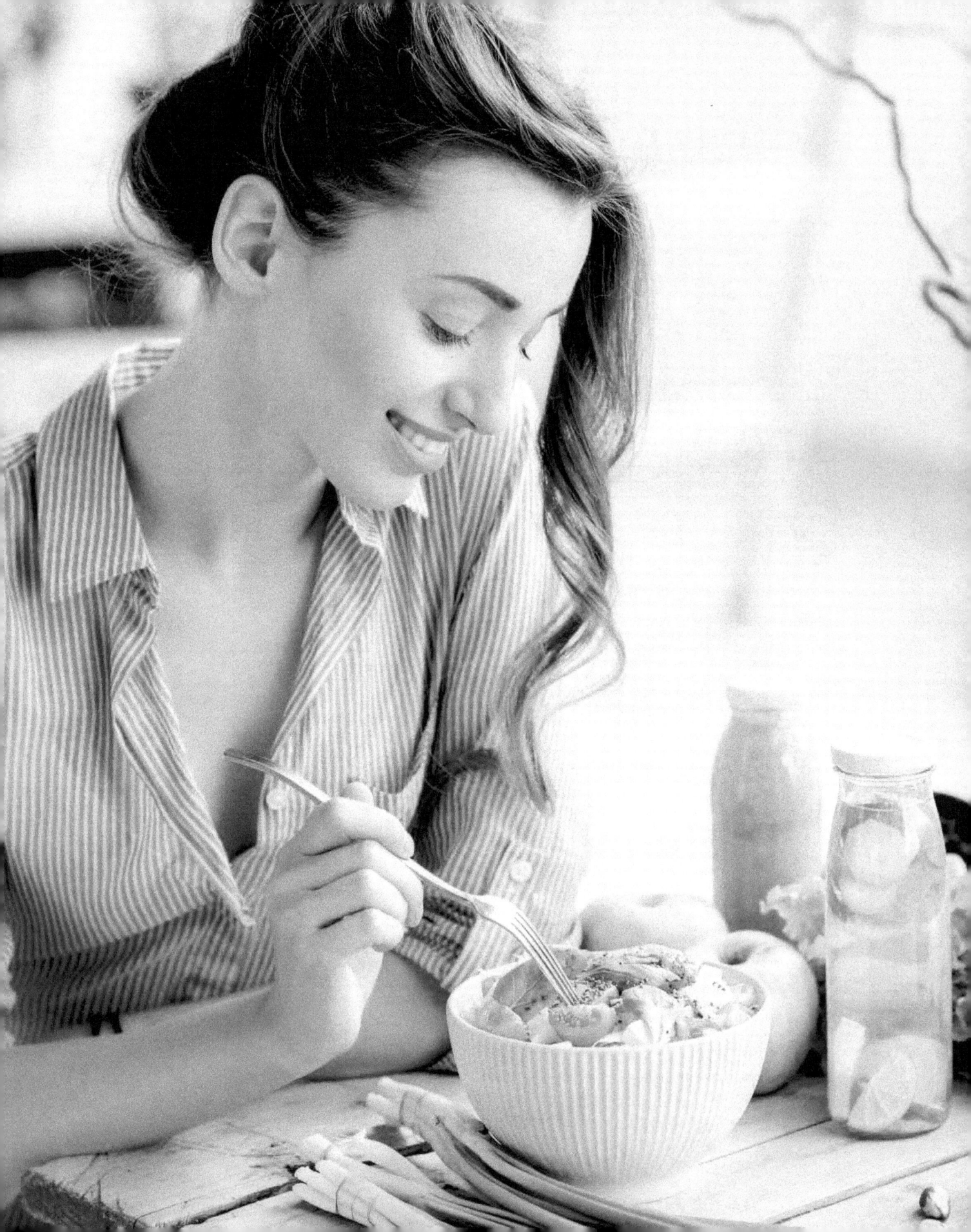

Conclusion

Keto foods provide a high per calorie amount of protein. This is important because the basal metabolic rate (the number of calories required daily for survival) is less for the aged. However, they still need the same amount of nutrients as the younger ones.

A person 50+ will find it much harder to live on junk foods than a teen or 20-something whose body is still resilient. This makes eating foods that are health-supporting and disease-fighting even more important for seniors. It can mean the difference between fully enjoying the golden years or wasting them in pain and agony.

Beginning the Keto diet can seem daunting at first, but you have all of the information you need to help you start! I hope you find the courage and motivation to follow your new lifestyle to experience all of the incredible benefits that come with the diet.

This diet plan isn't going to hinder you or limit you, so do your best to keep this in mind as you begin changing your lifestyle and adjusting your eating habits. Packed with good fats and plenty of protein, your body will go through a transformation as it works to see these things as energy. Before you know it, your body will have an automatically accessible reserve that you can utilize. Whether you need a boost of energy first thing in the morning or a second wind to keep you going throughout the day, this will be inside you.

As you take care of yourself through the next few years, you can feel great knowing that the Keto diet aligns with the anti-aging lifestyle that you seek. It keeps you looking great and feeling younger. Still, it also acts as a preventative barrier from various ailments and conditions. The body tends to weaken as you age. Keto helps to keep a shield up in front of it by giving you plenty of opportunities to burn energy and create muscle mass. Instead of taking the things that you need to feel great, Keto only takes what you have in abundance. This is how you will always end up feeling your best each day.

Keto is an adjustment, but it is one that will continue benefiting you for as long as you can keep it up. If you are ready to feel great and look great from the inside out, you can begin your Keto journey with the confidence that it is truly going to make a difference in your life. The natural signs of aging and hormonal imbalances of being a woman are not enough to hold you back when you are actively participating in a balanced Keto diet.

Change your life today and enjoy the many benefits of a Keto diet.

CPSIA information can be obtained
at www.ICGtesting.com
Printed in the USA
LVHW060531111120
671124LV00013B/332

9 781914 144103